£2.50

Statistics in Operation

Statistics in Operation

Winifred M. Castle
MD, MFCM, MBBS, MIS
Formerly Reader in Community Medicine,
University of Rhodesia

CHURCHILL LIVINGSTONE
EDINBURGH LONDON AND NEW YORK 1979

CHURCHILL LIVINGSTONE
Medical division of Longman Group Limited

Distributed in the United States of America by
Churchill Livingstone Inc., 19 West 44th Street, New York,
N.Y. 10036, and by associated companies,
branches and representatives throughout
the world.

First published 1979

ISBN 0 443 01951 7

British Library Cataloguing in Publication Data

Castle, Winifred Mary
Statistics in operation.
1. Mathematical statistics 2. Medical statistics
I. Title
519.5'02'461 QA276 78-41279

Printed in Great Britain by Bell & Bain, Glasgow

Preface

The purpose of this book is to provide workers in the medical sciences in particular, with a cheerful, non-mathematical elementary account of the use and abuse of the statistical approach.

As a practicing doctor you may be about to decide that any book about Statistics is not for you. If in your particular branch of medicine you never take chances and never read medical journals then you are right. Similarly if you are a capable academic steering your own clinical hunches over all the hurdles to a valid result, then side-step this book.

As a profession most of us would admit that we are forced to take chances and calculated risks. Therefore, there is a definite place in most aspects of medicine for an understanding of the science of odds or statistics. This book is directed at doctors and paramedicals who recognise that they take chances but who hate juggling with numbers. It is for those who skip articles in medical journals as soon as they see reference to a standard deviation - but then feel they should not have done so because they may be missing out on something of value. It is intended for doctors outside an academic environment who are keen to follow up one of their clinical hunches with an investigation. At best, I hope this book will make the use of numbers in medicine more interesting; at worst I hope it will protect you from their misuse.

The book was prompted originally by a comment in a review of my original programmed learning text-book *Statistics in Small Doses* - that the reader required supplementary material to put the whole subject into perspective. I agree, and in fact my medical students here have lectures as well as the prescribed text-book. This book is more or less the content of their lecture course. Over the years I have found that having persuaded the students to do 'sums' it is better to cut out the chatter. Similarly if you want students to listen to chatter it is better to lay off the sums. Consequently this book is not spoilt by arithmetic.

My lecture notes have developed over more years than I would wish to acknowledge. Most of the points have arisen in discussing medical research with my medical colleagues, postgraduate and undergraduate medical students and I am particularly grateful to those who remain my friends. I must have taken other points from different sources, the origins of which I have forgotten, but I am grateful.

The ideas were put into better English by Phillipa Christie, Gwen Livingstone and Aubrey Mitchell, to all of whom I am grateful. The drawings were prepared by Mrs Hilary Goldsmid and Mrs Joan Henry. Miss Fiona Hamilton and Mrs Mary Peters typed the final draft of the manuscript.

'I suppose the reason we have two ears is so we can listen to two people at the same time'. Two people in particular have given a lot of time and effort and 'it can be no dishonour to learn from others when they speak good sense'.

First, Mrs Daphne Russell of the University of Newcastle on Tyne suggested in particular the re-organisation of the text into its present form. In my view this has resulted in a substantial improvement. I am also grateful to her for the thoroughness with which she advised on an earlier script.

In particular, I would like to thank my teacher and friend of long standing, Professor David Cox of Imperial College. Of course, the really wise sentences are his! As busy as he was he willingly devoted much time, quiet good humour and patience. He spends himself ...

Having acknowledged the substantial contribution of so many you may be wondering where I fit into the scheme of things - why my name is on the cover! I organised and listened to everyone; mine were the scissors which cut earlier scripts and the sellotape which restuck them together; mine are any mistakes which remain and the responsibility for them.

1979 W.M.C.

Contents

Introduction
Statistics: Sense not sums

Man is a biped but fifty men are not a centipede.
G.K. Chesterton.

The reason we cannot simply add and subtract information about people is that people vary. Individuals not only look different; thankfully they also behave differently. To tackle the fact of variability a knowledge of statistics is needed. What do we mean by statistics?

Statistics originally dealt with state records, but it now incorporates a search behind bald statements in an attempt to find the truth. This is the bikini aspect of statistics - the exposed parts are interesting, but it is the concealed parts which are vital.

This quest for the truth has not always been considered important. Even today the social and academic status of the person speaking is of paramount importance in most people's assessment of what is said.

Bertrand Russell reminds us that when it was first proposed to establish laboratories at Cambridge University, Todhunter - the mathematician - objected that it was unnecessary for students to see experiments performed since the results could be vouched for by the teachers - all of them men of the highest character and many of them clergymen of the Church of England.

Using statistics we attempt to take an impartial look at the results of experiments in order to determine the probabilities of truth or untruth of any interesting hypothesis. By and large statisticians parallel the approach of English lawyers and assume a kind of statistical innocence regarding the truth of any new proposition until the evidence is such that its real effect is established 'beyond all reasonable doubt'.

A statistical analysis assesses the evidence, telling us how likely we are to be correct or incorrect in believing a new hypothesis is untrue. Gallileo said 'The aim of science is not to open a door to infinite wisdom but to set a limit to infinite error,' This is certainly true of the science of statistics.

Some of my own students have defined statistics as 'that product of the untalented sold by the unprincipled to the utterly bewildered'. A closer definition would be that statistics is a 'numbers game' - the application of common sense to the numerical facts of life. In medical practice we use statistical methods so that we are in a better position to act in the face of uncertainty. The qualified doctor, having spent six years learning how to follow up clinical hunches, then spends a lifetime developing the art of taking risks without being too obvious about it. Doctors in all specialities only do the best they can in a series of essentially uncertain situations. Even the important distinction between dead and not dead has become blurred medicolegally.

Although they do not gamble recklessly, physicians take a chance every time they prescribe a drug in that they can only believe it will do more good than harm. Surgeons talk openly about 'operation risks', not only with their medical colleagues, but actually with the patients and their relatives. 'Intervention' is a gambling term introduced by obstetricians. It means that the odds are stacked against a normal delivery and therefore they must decide to back either their forceps or vacuum extractors.

Outside the hospital the general practitioners follow their hunches all day. They speculate about whether a set of sumptoms are psychological, whether a particular girl is possibly pregnant, and so on. Meanwhile swivelling in their chairs the medical administrators weigh up different priorities - fortunately for them they bet with other people's money! The witchdoctors openly and unashamedly toss their bones. Are we not as a profession merely charging more and adding touches of sophistication to the same toss-the-bones princiiples?

Certainly we do not always follow our hunches without weighing up the evidence. The academic doctors, with their limited number of beds, have the time to work out some of the odds. Sitting astride their clinical hobby-horses like jockeys, they scurry to push their noses through the winning post - acceptance by the medical journals - before anybody else in their particular field. Spurred on by the drug companies, they quote odds to the general medical punters who are nearly always willing to listen - and then stake their bets.

The medical profession is a noble one. It does not allow this clinical race meeting to proceed without supervision. There is a course steward encouraging the academics to produce reasonable odds on the one hand and protecting the punter from foul play on the other. Although there are two sides to this official's task, they are closely inter-related. The principles involved in encouraging fair analyses are the same as those used to encourage the reader to recognise unfair ploys used by some writers in medical journals. To know how to barge is the first step towards realising when you are being barged. The gentleman here introduced, the course steward, without his racing guise, is the medical statistician. How does a medical statistician see the situation?

Numbers are put to good and bad use in medicine. With previous generations the distinction was probably less relevant than it is today. Quinine, until confusion arose over the bark of the Rubiaceaen tree, was obviously beneficial in the early treatment of malaria. Ether and chloroform had easily recognised effects. The Ayurvedic physicians in India knew about the sedative effect of the Rouwolfia plant long before more detailed study also highlighted the drug's hypotensive effect.

Medical research today does not generally leap forward in giant strides. Knowledge is usually inched forward by careful comparisons between different drugs or surgical methods. Perhaps Christian Barnard and other jockeys in his field did not particularly need a statistician at the time of their first few heart transplants. Nor, fortunately, do I at the moment require their services. However, the best surgical techniques, immunosuppressive regimes and cost benefits, if any, will only be discovered after extensive use of sophisticated statistical methods.

If statistics is therefore a necessary discipline in medicine today, it is unfortunate that doctors often seem to have such a bad reputation in this field so far as other scientific professions are concerned. Over the ages adaptations have been made by the statisticians to suit medical needs, but when medicine and statistics meet the result is usually, it is said, an unholy alliance rather than a happy marriage.

As one homosexual said to his pal as he saw a man and his wife fighting, 'There, I told you those mixed marriages never work'.

Perhaps the same could be said of many other fields of statistical application, but it is important that some sort of medicostatistical alliance should be made to work, and in my view some of the outside criticism is ill deserved. Agriculturalists and biologists can move cows from pasture to pasture and mate hamsters virtually at will in the course of their experiments. In contrast, doctors are often lucky to get a hospital bed at all, let alone borrow somebody elses for purposes of medical research, however worthwhile the results could prove to be. Medical ethics cannot be made the servant of science, and so many research doctors' hands are tied in practice in a way their critics do not appreciate.

I once attempted to assess the extent to which this outside criticism of doctors was justified. I decided to cast a medicostatistical eye over a selection of medical journals published inside and outside Africa. These were the first six editions published during 1970 of the *South African Medical Journal, Medical Journal of Zambia, Central African Journal of Medicine, Medical Proceedings, The Lancet, The British Medical Journal, The Journal of Obstetrics and Gynaecology of the British Commonwealth* and the *Journal of the American Medical Association.*

Altogether this gave a total of 48 editions incorporating 267 articles. Of these, 168 were either surveys or reports on drug trials, and used statistical methods. The other 37 per cent were narrative, mainly individual case reports. Although the journals considered do not perport to be representative of all medical literature they serve to illustrate the very substantial usage of statistical methods in medicine.

Astonishingly, the use of statistics is almost matched in practice by its misuse. I identified no less than 362 separate mistakes in the 168 articles which were statistically vulnerable, a figure which gives an average of over 2 errors per article. While it must be emphasised that this is the view of only one person, any other researcher repeating the exercise would also have shown that the problem was of considerable magnitude. The 362 errors do not describe the problem fully because only errors of detail were counted. No attempt was made to assess errors of basic approach.

In certain instances the errors discovered were very much worse than others; intentionally or not, some of the authors were not only liars but 'damned liars'. It was very evident that in some of the journals outside Africa the standard of lying was more subtle, in that by subtelty they appeared to make smaller untruths go further. However, since the most prevalent mistakes were common to all the journals, they need not be particularised, but rather considered as a whole.

Treatment of a medical complaint is always easier if causes of the problem are known, and with this in view, the 362 mistakes were classified. If the commonest statistical errors could be easily explained, medical authors could perhaps have their deficiencies remedied.

Reference to Table 1 shows that these three hundred and sixty-two errors all fell into one of twelve categories, with the majority falling into eight.

Only Categories 4, 9 and 12 may be described as requiring detailed statistical knowledge and these account for less than 14 per cent of the total.

The remaining mistakes are not difficult to understand but each and every one contributes to the bad reputation which the profession earns for itself.

I concluded after my survey that we doctors do seem to use statistics like drunken men a lamppost - for support rather than illumination - and that our shortcomings are not only due to failure to understand the mathematical recipes.

I admit that my impression is, but I have no proof, that the situation has tended to improve recently. There are still problems. Not only should we analyse our results better but there are the problems of finding the correct data to analyse and of drawing the correct conclusions on the evidence once the results are analysed. After all there are many ways of trying to answer the same medical research question, each of which may produce different sets of data, analyses and conclusions and the overall need is to reflect on which is the wisest method of organising a research project.

So there is much more to statistical abuse than dishonesty with arithmetic. Many 'lies, damned lies and statistics' one can recognise in others and can avoid oneself without resort to any numerical gymnastics.

Table 1 Classification of errors in 168 articles in the medical journals.

Rank	Category of mistake	Frequency
1	The wrong control group or no control group at all (where one was required)	60
2	Conclusions without evidence	56
3	Faulty diagrams and tables	46
4*	No significance test where one was indicated	44
5	Failure to quote significance test used or significance level attained	28
	Missing subjects not accounted for	28
7	Arithmetical errors	27
8	Ill-defined terminology or wrong term used	24
9*	Wrong significance test used	16
10	Negative findings incorrectly stated	14
11	Positive findings incorrectly stated	11
12*	Too many significance tests used	8
	Total	362

*Requiring detailed statistical knowledge.

What can we do to improve the situation? For a start we can try to stop any breakdown in communications between doctors and statisticians. The jargon often means different things to different groups. It is true that words such as 'bias' and 'significance' convey the same broad ideas to both groups, but the shades of meaning and implication still hidden are of fundamental importance.

Politically terms such as 'apartheid', 'communism' and 'one-man-one-vote' can be defined by different shades of political opinion. While the actual meaning of, for instance, 'one-man-one-vote' is straightforward, the political and ethical implications range in different people's eyes from moral perfection to economic chaos - not to mention the horror on the faces of the women's libbers who cry for one-ms-one-vote! The political interpretation of these terms is as vital as is their definition. Even when they are conversing in the same language I sometimes wonder whether politicians with different view-points really understand what the other side is talking about. I think the difficulty of interpretation is as acute in medical statistics as in politics and there is undoubtedly a great need for a medico-arithmetical settlement.

The implication of words such as 'significance' has to be conveyed without misunderstanding between research doctor and statistician. From them the proper meaning must be transmitted via the journals to the practising doctor. Each link in the chain must preserve the true message. Unfortunately, 'send reinforcements we're going to advance' intended at the beginning of the chain is all too often interpreted eventually as 'send 3/4d we're going to a dance'. So I shall avoid discussing stodgy definitions and talk about their interesting implications for, after all, articles in the journals are trying to convey a message rather than test knowledge.

There are other ways in which we could improve our professional front so far as statistics are concerned. Some doctors *refuse* to know anything about the subject and this should not be allowed. Admittedly many books with their heavy arithmetic and algebra, not to mention the Greek symbols, leave many doctors unresponsive even if they are keen to understand the principles. I will avoid falling into this trap while pointing a finger at the attitudes of the few who put up their shutters against statistics without trying to understand them. Some go even further than putting up their statistical shutters. From the security of their closed shops they then go on to hurl abuse at the subject. Medical statisticians, contrary to popular opinion, do not sit along the road of medical progress poking spokes in every passing wheel. As other sciences have advanced, so have the mathematical aspects of medicine. The doctor who thinks current statistics always demand large scale expensive and completely unpracticable experiments is out of date.

Doctors can also improve by seeking advice before they start a clinical trial if they suspect their ability to see the experiment through alone. Medical information is often very expensive and time consuming to collect and should not be wasted. Although statistics can now go a fair way towards fitting in with the practical aspects of clinical trials, the method of collecting the data can make or break it as far as analysis is concerned. Unfortunately very accurate information is no better than shoddy experimentation if it cannot be used. Every statistician I know would willingly perform the arithmetical contortions for a doctor who has taken care with suturing the medical and mathematical aspects initially.

The aim of this book is therefore to encourage the reader to apply common sense to the gambling aspects of medicine rather than to provide understanding of detailed statistical formula.

What is the best approach? The mistakes identified in the error-ridden journals previously mentioned could be explained in detail so that, hopefully, the reader could understand them and avoid making them in the future. Instead, we will use the same information to emphasise pitfalls as we chat about designing research projects.

We will discuss in turn the implications behind a list of ten questions which I use to organise my own thoughts while thinking or talking about research outlines.

The ten questions are these:

1. What exactly is the question we want to answer?
2. What are the main practical considerations?
3. What will we measure?
4. Who is going to do the work?
5. About whom are we talking?
6. Who will be measured?
7. How will the data be presented?
8. Shall we be able to answer our original question?
9. Shall we be able to interpret the answer?
10. So what?

This is the How? Who? What? and Why? in any research undertaking. The first point is that all ten questions should be answered in theory, as far as possible, before any of the practical work is started.

So often, halfway through the project the research worker discovers that his method is not comparable to somebody else's, an underlying assumption is incorrect, the control group is wrong, or some other anomaly has reared its ugly head. It is then difficult, if not impossible, to salvage any results for the effort. I know because it has happened to me and to nearly all my colleagues at some stage or another.

Without being mathematical, therefore, let us wander down the medical scientific research pathway; observation - hypothesis - experiment - conclusion. The initial observation is usually of a clinical nature, the rest of this book describes the other sections of the journey. Relax. Mathematics will honestly be kept to a minimum. It is more important that we use our lamp-posts correctly.

1. What exactly is the question we want to answer?

What's the use of running when you are on the wrong road?
W.G. Benham.

Many go wrong at the beginning because they are not clear in their own mind what exactly they are trying to do. It sometimes seems, even from the articles accepted for publication, that the research workers hoped that if they stirred much information for a sufficiently long time then something useful might turn up.

Just as it is important in teaching to decide one's aims and objectives before giving a lecture, so is it important in research to spell out fully and in a straightforward manner what exactly one is trying to do. Everything else hinges on this, because an ill-defined question can only produce an ill-defined answer.

What is the prevalence of neurosis in a given general practice? As it stands this question is not fully spelt out. Does the question only require the grand total for its answer? Is the work to involve a categorisation of patients into such as age, sex, marital status, race, socioeconomic and occupation groups? - a numerical as well as a nervous breakdown! If so, it is necessary to ask all these sub-questions at the beginning.

It is also important at the outset to decide whether symptoms and signs, duration of the disease, whether the disease is acute or chronic, and whether the case was previously known to the doctor or is newly diagnosed, are also going to require analysis.

One must beware of trying to do too much because most people are able to perform a small task more accurately than a large one. 'The dinosaur's eloquent lesson is that if some bigness is good, an over-abundance of bigness is not necessarily better'.

It is wise not to try to go too far, particularly with information which is difficult to measure accurately. For example, 'duration of neurosis' is difficult to assess, because it is not easy to pinpoint the exact onset unless the particular mental state was caused by social circumstances which changed suddenly.

Having fully defined the question the next problem is to define the terms used. Some readers may not be able to define the word 'prevalence' which is defined later in this book. One of the most difficult tasks is how to define the particular disease one is talking about. How would one define the word 'Neurosis'? Various possibilities spring to mind.

'The neurotic person knows that two and two make four but is terribly worried about it; the phychotic person knows that two and two make five and is perfectly happy about it.'

Then again it has been said that neurotics are those people who build castles in the air as opposed to psychotics who live in them. There would remain a problem even if all the doctors were to accept an arbitrary definition imposed on the term by some eminent doctor such as 'a disturbance of the mind in which the patient retains contact with reality'. Their impressions of when that definition had been complied with would all be totally different.

You may think that neurosis is a particularly amorphous term to define. This may be so but I once asked a group of medical practitioners to define the more specific term *hypertension*. No two individuals came up with exactly the same answer. For example, different allowance was made for the effect of age increase, duration of bed rest before taking the blood pressure and for other medical conditions such as pregnancy. Cecil and Loeb in their textbook of medicine use 70 lines to define hypertension. You may think it is not desirable to have a rigid dividing line for such conditions. In caring for an individual patient a wise physician will assess the condition on its merits. A systolic blood pressure of 182 in the clinical sense is no different from one of 180. Upper levels of normality as quoted by pathologists are only guidelines. However, in the research situation we do need to define the condition about which we report.

In passing, it is worth giving obstetricians not one of their own slaps on the back, but a pat on the back, because of all the branches of the medical profession they try to define most conscientiously their clinical conditions. Terms such as prematurity, antepartum haemorrhage and abortions are clearly signposted as well as more difficult conditions to define such as toxaemia.

Unfortunately in general the definition of a disease is usually difficult and full of 'ifs' and 'buts' even though the ifs and buts are given a more academic air and become 'usually' and 'ordinarily'. For example, Cecil and Loeb define influenza, that common disease, as 'an acute contagious disease that is usually attended by fever and prostration and is ordinarily benign in outcome'.

Of course all definitions are to a greater or lesser extent arbitrary. Nevertheless it is very important to be as precise as possible about what *you* mean. You should depart from generally accepted usage only for some very good reason.

It has been said that one can understand something of a profession by the jokes members tell about themselves. Certainly in the generation preceding this one the jokes doctors frequently told at gatherings were about psychiatric subjects. For example, two doctor frients met in the corridor of the hospital and one said to the other, 'You are all right; how am I?'. With an increasing emphasis on statistics this joke could be changed to the statisticians joke, 'How are you? How's your wife?' and his friend replying 'Compared with whom?'. Believe it or not, this story is relevant in defining a disease because if the findings in the current piece of research are to be contrasted with findings in previous studies this should be taken into account right at the beginning. Why? Because it must be decided at the outset to conform not only to their methodology but also to their definitions.

First, then, spell out the question; second, try not to do too much at once; third define the terms and in particular the disease being discussed; and finally decide at the outset whether you want your results to be comparable with those of A.N. Other.

2. What are the main practical considerations?

I had rather ride on an ass that carries me than a horse that throws me.
George Herbert.

We must ask ourselves now whether we think an answer to the fully defined question is feasible in practice. Have we sufficient time and money? Must we first seek authority from any board or committee? Do we need more clinical advice? Can we increase the willingness of patients to co-operate?

Many problems which have not been anticipated creep into a study and these can be cured before they precipitate a statistical emergency if, having decided how we are to plan the project, we organise a small dummy run. Such a pilot study is generally a good idea and it is an essential part of any major investigation. The idea is to make it as nearly like the finished article as possible - a dress rehersal - and the role of a pilot study will be mentioned later when we discuss techniques of measurement, the design of questionnaires and the numerical size of the groups we will study.

Another important point at this stage is ethics. Ethical decisions must be medical rather than mathematical but I believe the researcher has the responsibility to decide whether the possible discomfort of the patient is likely to be justified by a meaningful result. Statistically we are more directly concerned with whether the work is practicable and whether the most efficient use is being made of time and money.

There are three other statistical practicalities. First, do we need a control group, and if so which; second, are we to do an experiment or a survey and third, if we are to do a survey will we work forwards from now (prospectively) or retrospectively? These points are discussed now because 'the resolution to avoid evil is seldom framed till the evil is so far advanced as to make avoidance impossible' (Thomas Hardy).

Control or contrast groups

In my survey of the journals I found the control group was the stumbling block which tripped most doctors (Table 1).

I suppose this is partly because clinical medicine is full of controlling devices *not* related to the statisticians meaning of control. The gynaecologists spring to mind with their contraceptive pills to 'control' the population explosion. Surgeons are provided with an arsenal of artery forceps for 'controlling' haemorrhage. Physicians, more reticent in their wisdom, use hypotensive drugs, for example, to 'control' blood pressure.

Meanwhile radiologists try to keep radiographers out of mischief by asking them to take extra pictures which are often labelled 'controls'. This extra expenditure is necessary because X-ray controls are the yardstick against which boney conditions can be measured. It is in this sense that the statisticians also use the word 'control'. In the gambling aspects of medicine control groups are the yardsticks against which other groups are measured. Statistically the control group is the norm. For example if a group is to be given a new drug the control group may be given an inactive substance which looks the same as the drug - a placebo. The control group should always be as like the study group as possible except for the factor under review.

It is always necessary to have a control group? No, it is possible to describe a medical situation without it. For example, we can estimate that a particular death rate is such and such. The point is that this is usually of little use until there is some standard for comparison. Whenever a comparison is to be made some yardstick must be included. Sigmund Freud said, 'We are so made that we can derive intense enjoyment only from a contrast and very little from a state of things'.

No radiologist, if interested in the pathology of the left ankle, would get much, if any, help from an X-ray of a different patient's right ankle. It does seem, though that some editors of medical journals value control groups which bear little resemblance to a group under study. Indeed, if you are ever in the position where you cannot show what you want to show I suggest you try using the wrong control group. In the mental haze which is likely to be provoked you may well get away with the error.

You know the sort of thing: the death rate in the Army last year was less than in 'civvy street'. It is therefore safer to be in the Army than out of it! The figures are accurate, the conclusion is not. This is because the two groups are not comparable. The Army is made up of young men in good health. The civilian population includes infants, the old and the ill, all of whom in any case have a higher death rate. The conclusions have nothing to do with safety.

Remember that a difference can be large but it may not be meaningful if the comparison is not valid.

For example, in one article reviewed there was a study of the cardiographic effects of exercise. E.C.G. readings were taken of the heart condition of men who took regular exercise. A proper control group would have been men who took measurably less exercise in the same age group, and from the same background. The two readings could then have been compared and conclusions drawn as to whether those taking exercise were in better health than their counterparts. Of course, even with the correct control group one would still have to consider the possibility of those with poor hearts choosing not to exercise originally. We cannot determine from this study whether exercise improves E.C.G. recordings or a sound heart predisposes one to jogging. The cause and effect still cannot be separated.

However, in the particular research project a bad control was used. The results were compared with groups living in other countries and even in different age categories. Clearly the differences between the research project E.C.G. results and the so-called control groups could not be evaluated in terms of the effects of exercise. There are other possible explanations for the differences; different ages, different diets, different occupations and different climatic conditions as well as different genetic pools.

Of course it is quite possible to make comparisons between groups with different age distributions, but in order to do so effectively a certain allowance must be made for the difference, one allowance which can be made being the Age Standardised Mortality Rate. Its surgical cousin is the Age Corrected Survival Rate. They originate from a statistical gimmick whereby both sets of death experiences are applied separately to a single population so that there is no age discrepancy. Unfortunately these manoeuvres are unpopular in some circles because they replace genuine deaths with artificialities; corpses, with ghosts! 'Stone dead hath no fellow', quote the surgeons. However, without the artificialities of statistical standardisations and corrections it can be grossly misleading to compare Death Rates in two places and one surgeon's five-year survival rate with another's. One also sometimes has to standardise for time of year, social class, etc. For example in comparing two races it is as well to compare individuals of the same socioeconomic standing; otherwise a difference could be due to relative poverty rather than race.

In another article read during my review of the literature, a research project dealing with the effectiveness of antibacterial soap was discussed. The criterion for comparison was to be the incidence of skin infections in the group of soldiers using the antibacterial soap and the other group using the placebo - the insert unmedicated soap.

There should have been no difficulty in setting out comparisons. However, the two groups used were two different battalions in different parts of the war zone and having widely differing living conditions. The difference observed could therefore be as easily explained by the effects of the different living situations as by any difference in the effects of the two types of soap. The different soaps should have been allocated to soldiers living in the same circumstances.

Therefore the first decision is whether a control group is necessary in your project - it usually is. If so it must be as like the study group as possible. It must be selected at the same time as the study group or it is not acceptable. One of my colleagues was interested in the gut bacteria of children with measles. He contrasted his findings with those of a similar group of children without measles, but eighteen months later. It is as wrong to contrast people of the same age at different times (unless time is the factor under consideration) as it is to contrast people of different ages at the same time (unless age is the important factor).

It is, of course, much easier to criticise a control group used by somebody else than it is to select an acceptable one for yourself. This is particularly so within a hospital. Even those admitted on account of accidents cannot be accepted as being otherwise well. Accidents do not just happen and the deaf, the small, the stupid, the short sighted and the boozers must be at greater risk. The selection of a proper control group is difficult in hospital practice but it is of fundamental importance that we appreciate what it is we are seeking and the limitations of the control groups available.

Sometimes it is possible for a patient to act as his or her own control. For example the same people can be compared before and after treatment. Sometimes they can be given all of a series of treatments but then, of course the order in which they receive the treatments must be fairly allocated.

Experiments and surveys

One solution to the problem of selecting a control group is for the researcher to be the one to allocate a group of subjects either to the study group or the control before the subjects get the drug, diet, or factor under investigation, i.e., the 'treatment'. If this allocation is carried out fairly the groups will be comparable. This is the situation in must drug trials and because the research workers decide which subjects go into which study group it is called an 'experiment'.

In a 'survey' the subjects have already assigned themselves to different groups and the research workers only assess what is already present. One definition of the word survey in the dictionary is to 'behold from a commanding position' - such as a professorial chair! In medical research a survey is *not* a passive unplanned panoramic view of life in which the people go untouched - or it should not be! A surveyor is an investigator and a survey is different from uncontrolled routine data such as hospital statistics which have been collected for some other non-specific purpose.

A wit described an experiment as 'an interference with nature', and to the extent that a survey would then be an evaluation of unadulterated nature, the above definition is partially acceptable. But in a survey a patient may have experimental gadgets protruding from every conceivable (and non-conceivable) orifice with a highly academic team analysing every body juice - thus interfering markedly with nature - and yet this would still be a survey.

An example of a 'survey' was the exercise/E.C.G. study because the investigators had not decided which men would exercise. To 'experiment' the researcher would have divided a homogenous group of men into those who he required to exercise and those who would be required to sit and think - or just sit.

The difference between an experiment and a survey is important because it affects the conclusions which are possible. In an experiment in which the allocation is done fairly the control group initially will be comparable to the study group, any differences being only due to chance. Therefore if a significant difference is found at the end of an experiment it can be due to one of two alternatives, chance or the effect of the treatment. We will discuss later how to discriminate between these two.

In a survey the researcher compares one already selected group with some other control group. We have discussed the problems with selecting a control group in such circumstances. We can never be certain that there isn't a third alternative to explain differences seen, besides chance and the factor or disease we are considering. This third alternative is an unknown factor associated with the self selection of the study group.

Consider a survey on smoking and coronary artery disease. A significant association between smoking and the disease, if found at the end of the project, could have three possible explanations. It could be due to chance differences between the study and the control group and it could be due to smoking (the two alternatives of an experiment) but it could also be due to some other common factor - a particular psychological make-up, for example, may predispose both to smoking and coronary artery disease. There may be a genetic basis or a familial tendency to both. It is often unlikely that some other factor is to blame but the point is we can never be certain in a survey. This is especially so as the medical profession can only recognise the tip of the pathologico-psychological 'iceberg'.

Medical research needs surveys because it must deal with people who have already classified themselves into the group having a disease. They are useful in suggesting associations between factors and the disease, but remember the red herrings, and remember to plan them in the same detail as you would an experiment.

Prospective and retrospective surveys

A survey can be 'prospective' so that we look into the future or 'retrospective' so that we operate with regard to the past.

Retrospective work is so often the poorer relation that it has been called 'backward' in both senses of the word, i.e., looking backward and being inferior. Sometimes the information in retrospective surveys is taken from patient case notes in which event it is often unreliable because important factors have been omitted from some records. Perhaps the information has to be recalled by memory and this is particularly subject to bias.

Usually but not always retrospective studies contrast people with a particular disease with a control group without and a search is made for interesting features in their past. This is a case-control study. Where diseases are very rare the only feasible method of investigation may be a retrospective case control study and such surveys need not be condemned out of hand. The advantages and disadvantages of prospective and retrospective studies are highlighted in the following two studies.

One of the best known studies undertaken by Doll and Hill was a restrospective case-control study. They studied patients in hospital with cancer of the lung, matching each case by hospital, age and sex with another individual without cancer of the lung. Enquiries were made into past smoking habits - not an easy task as we will discuss later. A disadvantage of this type of study was the possibility of loss of reliability. Not only can people forget aspects of their smoking history - they can also possibly become biased by the time their medical condition is diagnosed. Also we are never too sure about the efficacy of the control group, particularly if it is research undertaken in winter, as in the wards there may have been many bronchitics who also smoked. Even if the control group is acceptable and is free from bias, nothing is learned about the relationship between other diseases and smoking.

So Doll and Hill later did a prospective study on smoking and lung cancer. They wrote to a 'cohort' or group of doctors enquiring about their smoking habits. These doctors were followed up for twenty years and their death notifications investigated. This type of prospective study is called a 'cohort' study which differs from a case-control because the people are initially divided on the basis of the factor, smoking in this instance, rather than on the presence of the disease. Being prospective the study was slower, and, being over two decades more difficult to administrate than the former retrospective study. The prospective results also required more careful analysis because, for example some smokers became non-smokers and vice versa. The advantages included gain in reliability and opportunity to investigate in the same survey an association between smoking and death from other disease such as coronary artery disease and chronic bronchitis. Finally because the doctors were originally grouped on the basis of their smoking habit, the actual risk associated with smoking could be calculated.

Notice that in both surveys useful information was gleaned but the gain in reliability of the prospective study statistically overshadows its inconvenience. In neither study could one conclude that smoking caused cancer of the lung. Both were only surveys and it is therefore impossible to eliminate the possibility of the intrusion of some unknown factor.

3. What will we measure?

> It's a good thing to have people size ye up wrong.
> Whin they've got ye'er measure ye'er in danger.
>
> *Finlay Peter Dunne.*

In the last chapter about practical statistical ideas control groups were discussed. A control group infers a comparison and the proper control group infers a valid comparison. In this chapter we see that the doctor must also be certain of what he is going to measure, what his criteria will be, what characteristics he will use to judge between the two or more groups he proposes to contrast.

Such criteria should be first, clearly defined; second, objective rather than subjective; third, quantitative rather than qualitative, fourth, sufficiently precise and last, limited in scope.

a. *Clearly defined*

Emphasis has already been placed on the fact that the original question and the diseases themselves should be clearly defined. It is equally true that if research interest is centred on the blood pressure of particular patients the procedure for taking the blood pressure must also be strictly defined. The conditions for taking the blood pressure must be made uniform over the duration of the project, otherwise the comparisons are worthless.

Do we need to record the diastolic pressure when the sound changes as in Britain or when it disappears as in America? How long must the patient rest beforehand? Can he be sitting or must he be lying? Will we ignore the first reading or the reading on the first visit when the subject may be particularly tense? We must spell out the method.

b. *Objective*

The subjects of the medical research have their own opinions or symptoms which are, by definition, subjective. The researcher will find that objective criteria are usually more reliable. Medical histories given by patients are useful but physical signs objectively elicited by the doctor, the pathologists reports, the findings which actually exist are more conclusive clinically and statistically.

Whenever obtainable, objective results should be preferred to subjective opinions. The story is told about an American survey which was once carried out to investigate the magazines read. Questions had been asked in all sorts of neighbourhoods all round the country. When the results were tabulated and analysed it appeared that a great many people loved *Harper's Magazine* and not many read *True Story*. Now there were publishers' figures around at that time that showed very clearly that *True Story* had a bigger circulation in millions than *Harper's* had in hundreds of thousands. The only reasonable conclusion was that a good many respondents (as people are called when they answer such a question) had not told the truth. About all the survey had uncovered was, more or less, an amount of snobbery.

Similarly the next time you read that the number of codeins eaten average 1,02 per day per student while the number of dagga cigarettes average 5,45 per day, ask the question, 'How can anyone have found out such a thing?' How valid were the replies? Were the respondents being honest? Not that I think people always lie. Bertrand Russell made much of such paradoxes as 'X says that everything he says is untrue. Is he telling the truth?'

Deliberate lying is only one source of error. People may be too careful not to give you a biased answer, which is often as disastrous. Of course, 'there is one sure way to find out if a man is honest and that is to ask him. If he says he is honest you know he is crooked.' (Groucho Marx). Nevertheless, the aim here is to make use of information gleaned by an observer rather than depend on the symptoms and opinions reported by the subject.

This is not always possible, of course. Sometimes reliance has to be placed on subjective information drawn from a patient. An example is a drug trial dealing with the treatment of migraine. The effectiveness or otherwise of the drug is dependent upon the subjective evaluation of the headaches of those included in the experiment. All patients in such subjective drug trials should receive some treatment, and one method of getting fairer results is to ensure that the patient is unaware of the treatment being given. The experiment would be 'blind' (to use the technical jargon). To take this one step further we could ensure that the doctor evaluating the response was also unaware of the particular treatment being given to the patient at that time (a 'double blind' trial).

This also brings up the problem of side effects in a drug trial. One possibility is to write the question on individual cards, shuffle the pack and let the patients answer each one for themselves. This does away with the order of the questions and intonation of the voice because there are problems in asking the question as well as interpreting the answer and both of these factors, the order and the intonation, may affect the validity of the responses given.

This brings us to the use - and misuse! - of a formal list of questions as used in a questionnaire. I always try to avoid questionnaires like the plague because if the questions are at all ambiguous the answers are meaningless and it is extremely difficult to ask questions that are not ambiguous. Many medical investigators underestimate the problem. They are clear in their own mind what the question means - but is the respondent? Are we right to assume that 'length of residence' will be given in years and months and not feet and inches?

You know the sort of question: 'Do you add a lot of salt to your food?' 'Do you prefer your food hot?' 'Do you cough?' I cannot honestly answer these questions about myself and it is as well to try your questionnaire initially on yourself. Then try a small group of your colleagues - particularly the 'nitpickers'.

Even in the true-false type of final examination paper we read 'Not rare complications of mumps include' and the bewildered student comments 'Do you want common or non-existent complications?' 'Examinations are formidable to the best prepared for the greatest fool can ask more than the wisest man can answer'. Negative questions are confusing in general and should not be included in examinations or in questionnaires. Qualifying adverbs such as 'usually', 'sometimes', 'rarely', 'commonly', and 'occasionally' also make the questions ambiguous. The difference between 'never' and 'nearly never' may be clear-cut to a virgin, but when does 'nearly never' become 'hardly ever'?.

With the best will in the world it is difficult to ask questions which are so unambiguous that the meaning of the responses is clear. Yet sometimes questionnaires and opinions are needed and the only further advice that I can give is to use a pilot study and write the code to the answers at the same time as you construct the questions.

A first attempt may look like this:

Currently you smoke:

More than 60 cigarettes on average per day	☐
50 - 60 cigarettes on average per day	☐
40 - 50 cigarettes on average per day	☐
30 - 40 cigarettes on average per day	☐
20 - 30 cigarettes on average per day	☐
10 - 20 cigarettes on average per day	☐
0 - 10 cigarettes on average per day	☐

Sorry, there are the men who smoke exactly 10 or 20 or 30 etc., on average per day. Which box do they tick? Let's start again.

Currently you smoke:

More than 60 cigarettes on average per day	☐
50 - 59 cigarettes on average per day	☐
40 - 49 cigarettes on average per day	☐
30 - 39 cigarettes on average per day	☐
20 - 29 cigarettes on average per day	☐
10 - 19 cigarettes on average per day	☐
0 - 9 cigarettes on average per day	☐

You may prefer to ask the subjects to state 'the total number of cigarettes they smoked in the last 2 days'. Even then people may smoke more cigarettes at the weekend, so a questionnaire completed on a Monday may differ from one completed on a Wednesday.

Suffice it to say that the design of questionnaires for use in medical research is always difficult. Even the instructions can be ambiguous, as was found recently by a dental colleague who distributed a questionnaire about oral hygene to junior school children. The children were instructed to 'Draw a tick in the box next to the right answer.' One child did as he was told!

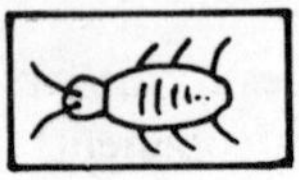

c. *Quantitative measurements*

We have decided to aim for objective results - things which we can see really exist. It is better that we choose objective criteria which we can actually *measure.* Wherever possible record an actual quantity, a figure, for each person investigated.

To categorise people as anaemic or not anaemic is technically called using qualitative information, results which only place people into categories on the basis of their having or not having that particular quality or charactistic. It is better to record the size or magnitude of the condition such as the quantity or level of haemoglobin. While it is true that we must define 'hypertension' if we are referring to hypertensive patients, it is wasteful to make no distinction in the hypertensive category between a blood pressure of 150/100 and 200/150 in recording results. It is surprising how many doctors throw away information by choosing only to divide patients into groups on the basis of quantitative results. It is not so important to note whether the girl is weaving a normal or a miniskirt - what is important is just how mini?

Scoring + or − on the basis of a mathematically ill-chosen dividing point may be disastrous if done at the recording stage. It may (or may not) be enough to analyse it qualitatively later. In the light of the data it is possible to choose cut off points which separate, for example, the top half from the bottom and this distinction may be useful in analysis. Quantitative results are usually grouped before diagrams are drawn. What is wrong is to throw away this detail of measurement at the recording stage.

We must decide whether the information is being used with maximum efficiency. I once delivered a paper concerning bilharzia and intelligence at a symposium. We were interested to see whether those children with bilharzia had a lower I.Q. than those clear of the disease. This is a qualitative criterion so far as the disease is concerned, the children being classed as either having the disease or being free. The paper was rightly criticised for failing to use the information more efficiently and in a quantitative manner. To do this we could have used the egg counts in those with bilharzia to indicate the severity of the disease.

Similarly with examination results there is more information in the quantitative score, 5 per cent., than in the qualitative grouping 'Fail' - the candidate may not agree.

d. *Sufficiently precise*

The point just made about wasting information must not be confused with making measurements too detailed. Groucho Marx said 'Either he's dead or my watch has stopped'. Although great emphasis has been placed on the necessity for a clear specification of criteria and a preference for quantitative measurements there is also the danger that information collected can become too detailed or too costly. There is a need for economy in the depth of the investigation. Money has already been mentioned and therefore the research worker should be sure, before embarking on an expensive and difficult exercise, that there is not some other quite simple clinical test which would prove adequate.

There is the story of the Social Medicine Examination question where students were asked to design a survey to screen for unsuspected diabetes. Incredibly, some students seriously suggested undertaking thousands of glucose tolerance tests, by post! 'It's just as unpleasant to get more than you bargain for as to get less.'

e. *Limited in scope*

Remember the old adage that 'if something can possibly go wrong it will'.

The previous point was not to dig too deep. The final point is not to spread your criteria too wide. The more clever we try to be, the greater the chance of error.

Collect only what is necessary after fully answering the question: 'What exactly are we trying to find out?' In general, only collect what you are going to use. This is also true for those doctors with computer services freely available! The more information that has to be obtained the more room is there for error, and therefore the less reliable the whole picture becomes. If a great deal of information is collected in a hurry the value of any individual reading or testimony may not be very reliable.

4. Who is going to do the work?

Those who believe they are exclusivily in the right are generally those who achieve something.

Aldous Huxley

The best answer to the above question is in my opinion yourself, i.e., the person most interested. The more people there are involved not only the greater the likelihood of things going wrong in general but the greater the problem of interobserver variation. Whenever more than one person is involved in laboratory analyses the taking of blood pressure readings, the coding of information from questionnaires and particularly in collating information from medical case histories, the answers will vary amongst those doing the work. The fewer 'those' are the more clearly defined will be the results.

Some would argue that, for example, with the coding of subjective opinions the researcher will often find it more difficult than an outsider to remain neutral. The researcher is liable to unconscious bias. My own view is that the outsider would probably also be aware of the answer hoped for and could also be vulnerable to unconscious bias. Presumably the researcher if undertaking the research at all is seeking the truth and my own view is that he or she should do the work. There is a Spanish proverb: 'If you want good service - serve yourself'.

Sometimes it is not possible for the director of the research to undertake all the work. If helpers are needed then a director should try to think of the factors which would make them better helpers. These include training, supervision and, in particular, motivation. If a technician has not only an interest shown in his work but also the opportunity to discuss with the supervisor the purpose and direction of the findings, he will usually be more enthusiastic about the way he goes about it.

A statistician can design a survey or experiment so that it is possible to allow for interobserver variation. These statistical methods are often used with biochemical data and in this situation it could be argued that it is better to use more than one technician.

Particularly in studying 'rare' diseases one has to acknowledge a place for very large co-operative trials. It may be impossible for doctors in one place to collect enough data to be of use in investigating factors affecting a cure rate. These co-operative studies seem essential but they do obviously raise major problems of standardisation of experimental techniques, etc. that can be largely bypassed in a 1-man band.

5. About whom are we talking?

> When schemes are laid in advance, it is surprising how often the circumstances fit in with them.
>
> *Sir William Osler*

The early volumes of the *Journal of the Royal Statistical Society* highlighted the hazards faced by medical pioneers when they were intent on evaluating entire populations. Their task was impossibly hard, standards inevitably fell and, partly because many workers must have been involved in collecting the information their results must have been unreliable.

What do we mean by a 'population' in a statistical sense? It is not necessarily a mass of people living in one neighbourhood. A population is the entire group about which some specific piece of research information is required. It is the subject of the experiment or the survey. It must be fully defined according to two main principles. In the first place the definition should be appropriate and in the second the definition must be foolproof.

A psychiatrist reported once that everyone was neurotic. Apart from the fact that such abuse of the word 'neurotic' destroys its meaning, the psychiatrist was presumably only talking about his patients. If a psychiatrist asks a man how he is, he does not often get the answer, 'Normal, thanks'. His population is inappropriate, as it often is in medical surveys, because the psychiatrist, of necessity, is basing his observations on a few patients and yet what is required is information about people in general.

My professor once calculated a rate for twinning in an up-to-date African central maternity hospital equipped for difficult obstetric deliveries which could not afford to admit the so-called 'normal' deliveries. Using this rate as its authority one textbook in genetics mistakenly stated that the area in which the hospital was situated had one of the highest twinning birth rates in the world and went on to discuss possible reasons.

You may conclude that Sch ... (by you know who) is beyond reasonable doubt associated with gout in your wards, but does this necessarily mean that all people who drink it are liable to gout? My advice to the research worker is to stick to discussing the population of patients in his ward only and to make this very clear. There will be plenty of readers who will still think he is discussing everybody. My advice to the reader of the research is to look as carefully at whom the doctor is describing as at the conclusions he draws. After all, what the butler saw was possibly interesting - but whom the butler saw was presumably more important! If the situation is not appropriate - the people must be!

We must as fully define the population we are talking about as initially we defined the question which we intended to answer and the terms used such as the diagnosis. A medical administrator may wish to survey trauma caused by motor accidents, perhaps with special regard to seat belts. The population in this instance consists of motor accident cases but these must be further defined. It must be decided whether it is meaningful to include pedestrians involved in accidents, cyclists, victims of trains hitting cars, etc. If it is, then these should not be excluded from the population to be sampled.

So that we can interpret the results properly, anyone involved in gathering information for the survey must know with certainty whether a particular road accident case should be included or excluded. The terms of reference for the survey population must have been clearly, even if pedantically, defined.

Some ambitious British medical school dean may have set himself the task, perhaps, of investigating medical opinion on some facet of medical education in one of the new medical schools. You might expect the population in this instance to be doctors in Britain. But would it? How would the population be defined? It would have to be decided whether, in the first place, there was a sufficient range of interests represented in those giving the opinions. Would Northern Ireland be included as part of Britain, for example, or would this depend on whether the people in charge of the survey believed in the wearing of the green? Would registered doctors generally be included, both those who are working and those who are not (this latter referring, naturally, to those who have retired rather than to those who boast a high leisure preference)? Should doctors practising inside, but trained outside, Britain be included in the survey and doctors trained in Britain but practising elsewhere? Or housemen? Or women? (notwithstanding the fact that the survey might primarily be read by a male chauvinist society.) Having made all these decisions, our population is finally defined but until this is done we cannot be sure to whom the conclusions refer and we cannot be sure how reliable our sampling method is likely to be.

And now, who are the guinea pigs going to be?

6. Whom exactly will we measure?

> I can stand brute force but brute reason is quite unbearable. There is something unfair about its use. It is hitting below the intellect.
>
> *Oscar Wilde*

At this stage of planning our research project we discuss some of the implications of sampling - of choosing a smaller group from within the defined population. A sample is used to estimate particular characteristics of the population, but because it is only a part it is only a shadow of the true population picture.

This is why sampling, however well chosen the method, always introduces a source of error. Sometimes this error is large enough to lead to a totally erroneous conclusion. During the course of one British general election all the opinion polls except one taken just before the polling day predicted a win for the Labour Party, basing their information on selected samples. The Conservative Party was successful with a fairly convincing majority although it is thought that many 'floating voters' changed their view just before the election.

In reviewing medical literature in depth it is often difficult to disentangle articles which report opposite conclusions - different views of the same picture. If we can assume that people are being honest in their publications, the most likely source of the controversy is in their choice of defined population or sampling method - although even with the same sampling method applied to a similar population it is possible but unlikely that conclusions will differ.

Often sampling cannot be avoided. At times, in clinical medicine it is the only method which can be used - in blood sampling, for example: more so when you are on the giving end of the needle than the person doing the testing. When the population is large and obtaining information about every member of that population is not possible, sampling cannot be avoided.

Ethics demand that a patient must be no worse off during a research project than he would be in the hands of a capable doctor and not taking part in the study. Within these constraints the medical profession owes it to society to make its conslusions valid. Their samples should, like a good photograph, provide a reliable image of the particular population. Just as a surgeon tries to make his biopsy specimen the best practical image of the organ, so the medical statistician tries to make his sample the best practical image of the population.

With a biopsy there is conflict between the reliable big slice the pathologists would like from the centre of the disease process and the convenient little slice from the periphery that medical students, if not the clinicians themselves, would wish to submit. So in sampling there is this reliability versus convenience battle. A good sample must be precise, and therefore a reasonable size; it must be unbiased or on-target, and it should be convenient to handle in practice. Often in life the wrong way seems the most reasonable. (Eating meat with your fingers is one example). Certainly this is true in so far as sampling is concerned. The most convenient samples are usually small but are therefore imprecise and are sampled badly and are therefore biased. A compromise has to be made between convenience and the other requirements of good sampling. What we gain on the unbiased and reasonably large swings, we usually lose on the roundabouts of easy administration.

Even in the most competent statistical shoes the step from talking about a sample to predicting about a population is as hazardous as is the step from talking about love to actually proposing. The sample is the major battleground of medicine and statistics. As a medically qualified statistician it makes me schizoid. My statistical left hand covets the biometrician's trump card, 'random mating', whereas my medical right hand demands a more conservative if not down-right prudish medical compromise. Perhaps the era of the promiscuous society will bring some relief! Even today the situation is not hopeless; a medico-statistical divorce is not inevitable, because in my experience there is always room for some compromise.

Two factors have to be decided: (a) What methods should be employed in selecting the guinea pigs? and (b) how many guinea pigs should the sample include?

a. *What sampling method?*

Basically, in our selection of a sampling method we are trying to avoid two types of error: bias and random error.

Statistically, *bias,* is a systematic error that would persist however large an investigation became and however many times the exercise were to be repeated using that particular sampling method. It results from an unfair method of choosing a sample. It is particularly a problem in surveys where it is often difficult in practice to devise a completely fair method of selecting individuals from an existing population. With such a biased sampling method the results are off-target and these methods should be avoided wherever possible.

With an unbiased sampling method the results are not exactly on-target. The *random error* remains. This is so even in an experiment where the population is fairly well fixed by the patients who are available and the problem is only one of dividing the population fairly into different samples.

If it is arranged so that every individual is equally likely to be assigned to any group this means that *on average* there would be no intrinsic difference between the different groups. However, this ideal situation where the sample gives an unbiased estimate - measures the accurate difference between the treatment groups and the control - only applies in theory and on average. For any particular set of samples in practice there is bound to be some difference between the groups just due to chance. In any particular instance sampling, even fair sampling, introduces an error - the random error. The random error becomes smaller as the investigation increases in size.

Random sampling methods

The concept of the random error divides sampling methods into two groups; the random or probability group on the one hand and the non random. The former group are basically fair, more reliable, but they are generally less convenient. They are more reliable because they are not biased in the statistical sense just described and using random sampling methods we are able to estimate the size of the random error on average. This measure of the size of the random error in the long run is called the standard error. Random sampling methods are generally less convenient in surveys than non random sampling methods because their basic requirement, before selecting a sample, is a complete list, in effect, of every member of the defined population.

Let us consider three different random sampling methods to see how they work out in practice - the simple random sample, the stratified random sample and the cluster sample. The implications are similar whether we are discussing the random allocation of treatments in designing experiments or the selection of individuals from a population in a survey even though the purpose is different. In my opinion doctors are more *au fait* with sampling in relation to experiments such as drug trials. Therefore we will concentrate more on a discussion of sampling from a population in a survey situation.

1. *The simple random sample*

This sampling method is the one most often quoted in theory. A simple random sample is one, by definition, into which each individual in the population has an equal chance of selection. Suppose we wanted to draw a sample of doctors in our survey of medical opinion about some facet of medical education. Remember we defined fully the population to be sampled and first of all, the doctors in the population must be listed. Next we would draw the names, or the number related to the name using a completely fair method, such as out of the boot of a Rolls Royce or by using a table of random numbers. In fact we would run a statistical lottery or a raffle to decide whom to include. To do so we would have to have complete knowledge of the population in the survey and this is the inconvenient part of a random sample. Certainly having availed ourselves of a complete list of the population it would not be a good idea to use a non random method.

The random sample has been called the 'statistical insurance against bias' but as already explained there is still the problem of the random error in any individual random sample. Any specific random sample may be unreliable because the one in a million chance does occur, even if *only* once in a million times. It is a possibility, though remote, that our noble profession's views would be represented entirely by the country's ENT surgeons - or perhaps worse, their anatomical neighbours, the thoracic surgeons! Therefore any particular simple random sample may give a result which is far from on-target.

It is interesting to ponder whether the dean would allow such an off beam sample of doctors as the one mentioned to stand or whether he would statistically err by putting all the names back and starting again, pretending such misfortune had not struck. Jonathan Swift said, 'I must complain the cards are ill-shuffled till I have a good hand'. Fortunately, I personally have not yet had such a decision to make! In simple random sampling with replacement in a survey if the same name is selected for inclusion in the same sample more than once, that person would be included more than once in theory, but few people would do this in practice.

The advantage of the simple random sample are that it is a fair method; on average the result would be on-target or unbiased even if in an individual simple random the result may be off target (due to random error). We can calculate the amount by which all possible simple random samples of that particular size and from that particular population are likely to vary by chance and the arithmetic to do this is easy to perform. Most statistical tests are based on the assumption that a sample is random.

One big disadvantage of the simple random sample - all random samples in surveys - is that up to date lists of populations are required. Another is that missing results are a bigger nuisance in random samples than in non random samples. This is because in the statistical sense that bias is a systematic error due to unfair sampling methods, random samples are free from bias so long as there are no missing results. We are never sure whether missing results are introducing a source of bias so we have lost the main advantage of choosing a random sampling method. If the method of sampling is non random we are forced, anyway, to accept the possibility that the samples are biased and that we are unable to estimate the magnitude of this bias problem.

We have already seen that a particular simple random sample can be way off beam. This problem is diminished by using the following random sampling method.

2. *The stratified random sample*

This sampling method is generally more reliable than the simple random sample but is even more inconvenient.

With foresight the problem of the ENT bias in our simple random sample of doctors could have been avoided by taking instead of a simple random sample a stratified random sample. This is more inconvenient in that each doctor would initially have to be stratified according to his or her speciality, e.g.:

Dr. L.S.D.	Psychiatrist
Dr. B.P.	Physician
Mr. L.P.	Neurosurgeon
Prof. R.A.T.	Academic
Mr. P.V.	Gynaecologist, etc.

A random sample would then be drawn within each stratum or speciality as the name of the method suggests, so that the different specialities would be represented in the final sample. If we considered the views of the G.P.s to be most relevant to our particular topic, there is nothing to stop us drawing a larger proportion from this stratum, although the subsequent arithmetic is slightly more involved if the proportion varies between strata. If the factors deciding the strata are relevant to the point under review, this stratified random sample is the most reliable of all. It has the major further benefit that as a by-product we could easily subsequently compare and contrast the views between the different specialities. Of course we could do this with the simple random sample although we might find some specialities were poorly represented (or in extreme cases totally absent). The main disadvantages in this most reliable sampling method of all are that it is administratively more difficult and if there are varying proportions the arithmetic becomes more involved. However in allocating treatment in an experiment using stratified random methods such as in drug trials we could for example, stratify for severity of the disease so that this factor could be studied in the analysis of the data.

3. *The cluster sample*

If members of the population in a survey are widely spread (communications-wise) the cluster sample is often the most reliable per unit cost. It would rarely be used in surveys inside the hospital wards or in experiments. However, if we had needed to visit our sampled doctors once we had selected their names in our survey of medical opinion, we would have made life easier for ourselves if we had drawn a cluster sample. How does a cluster sample fit into the random sample family? Before sampling we would group the doctors by practices. Each group, or 'cluster' of doctors would then be subjected to a random sampling procedure. Once a particular cluster had been selected, every doctor who was a member of the cluster would be included in the sample. This method could be used geographically where a map of the area could be gridded and the people in the randomly chosen small areas evaluated. In fact, it is a simple random sample but here the unit sampled is not an individual but a defined cluster of individuals. The arithmetic must be adjusted accordingly.

Non random sampling methods

In experiments such as drug trials where the patients are allocated randomly to treatment groups the differences measured may be due to random error or to the effects of the treatment. We can use tests of statistical significance to calculate how likely the difference is due to the random error, chance. The following group of sampling methods are non random. To apply significance tests without randomness is rather like treating disease X, which is more or less similar to disease Y, as though it was disease Y. We all do it but it is not without considerable risks so far as the outcome is concerned.

Life is not much fun if everything a person wants is either 'illegal, immoral or fattening'. Medical statistics is not much fun either if everything the article tells you is either incorrect, unethical or subject to error. So far this may be the impression this book is creating - to some extent it is the aim of this book.

We have discussed random sampling methods and have found them more or less reliable but inconvenient in medical surveys. We have decided that we prefer them to non random sampling methods. What is the positive side of non random sampling methods? By and large their convenience - they do not require the complete enumeration of the population. They are not even always unreliable. Their problem is that there is no measure of their unreliability. We can never be sure that they hit the nail on the head or whether they are systematically way off beam or biased.

As the actress must have said to the bishop, 'Let us take a short walk in the dark!' Let us think about three of the non random sampling procedures we encounter in medical journals - the systematic sample, volunteers and what may be called the haphazard sampling methods. Usually, but not always, they are used in survey work rather than in experiments.

1. *The systematic sample*

The systematic sample, as its name implies, is one in which say every fortieth patient either attending a surgery or being admitted to hospital is systematically included into the sample. It is the best of the non random methods. The good news is that the method is convenient and can be very representative. Now for the bad news. We are unable to say whether or not the sample is biased on account of its 'Achilles Heel', periodicity. The best way of explaining this is to draw on the example of going down a street and choosing every twentieth house. By coincidence it might so happen that every twentieth house (or every fortieth house) was on a street corner, standing in a larger garden than the rest of the houses in that particular road. Hence periodicity - a systematic error which biases the results. Every twentieth bed in the hospital may be nearer the ward sister's door with a patient nearer death's door. The danger of periodicity is that it can sneak in unnoticed, whether it be periodicity in place or in time. In a general practice every fortieth patient may tend to come towards the end of the day and include a higher proportion of businessmen or early in the morning and tend to be mothers of young children. Periodicity may not be a real factor in medical surveys but we can never be sure with the systematic sample. Even in a drug trial an alert sister may indulge in overt bias as she may have already decided which treatment she prefers and may negotiate the candidates for admission accordingly. This problem is counteracted, of course, not only by allocating treatment to the patients using random numbers, but also by running the experiment double blind.

2. *Volunteers*

Many medical surveys outside the hospital environment are based on a sample of volunteers. Of course all people in all medical research projects are required to state their willingness to participate; by volunteers we mean those who offer themselves without being specifically invited. (Like the actress?) There are major snags in interpreting results based on a sample of volunteers.

Imagine we want to estimate the average earnings of graduates of St. Thomas's Hospital inside as well as outside the British National Health Service. This may be for comparison with graduates from another medical school.

Doctors may be asked to volunteer the information by a general request in St. Thomas's Hospital magazine. We may receive a number of replies and could calculate the average income to be £15000! Does this mean that the average income of St. Thomas's graduates is, in fact, £15000? Of course not.

Who would reply to such a request? We might expect a higher proportion of the big income earners, the drug company directors, the top civil servants, any medical pop signers and the popular medical novelists. The majority of St. Thomas's doctors who would appear in *Who's Who* would be inclined to respond and in fact if they forgot to reply the people running the survey would probably realise they were missing and chase them up. Now what about the tramps, the alcoholics, or even junior University lecturers, people of whom it would take two or three or more to add up to an annual earning of £15000? Who are the people who would sling the questionnaire into the nearest wastepaper basket? - assuming their finances ran to such a luxury. It is a fair guess that even some graduates of St. Thomas's are just not making enough money to brag about. They are like the story of the little fellow who found a note clipped to his first pay cheque suggesting that the amount of his salary be considered confidential and not material for the inter-change of office gossip. 'Don't worry', he is said to have told the boss, 'I am just as ashamed of it as you are'.

On the other hand, if people were asked to volunteer the same information for purposes of a pay claim we may see an entirely different group coming forward. The motivation would be different and the moral of the volunteer story is that we do not really know much about what motivates a particular individual to volunteer.

I am the first to admit that medical surveys need volunteers. In investigating levels of coronary artery disease risk factors in relation of affluence we would have to study volunteers unless we had exhaustive information about residents in an area and their social status. The point is that we just do not know whether those volunteering to take part are motivated by the suspicion that they are at particular risk.

3. *The haphazard sample*

Many doctors inside the hospital seem to think that the completely haphazard or 'willy-nilly' sample is the same as the random sample. Some call them such - some editors of medical journals allow them to! You know the sort of thing - the 'I walked into the ward and chose X new admissions not knowing their diagnosis' type of control sample.

We now know that the simple random sample is the result of a very specific sampling proceedure. Random samples do not just happen - like any lottery - they have to be organised. I am not saying that medical research workers choose biased haphazard samples deliberately. We suspect that they often try to compensate for this possibility and end up leaning in the opposite direction.

Indeed, haphazard non random samples are not forced to be biased. Their chief snag is that we are in no way able to estimate the probability of bias having crept in - we are unaware whether we have cheated significantly or not.

Remember the rhyme:

Thou shalt not steal, an empty feat
When it's so lucrative to cheat.

We are unable to estimate how biased they are likely to be even when they are given an intellectual air by being served as a quota sample. This is used politically rather than medically and it occurs when a given number of people in different categories are chosen subjectively. For example, if we wanted an opinion on medical school curricula we could ask so many surgeons, so many physicians and so many obstetricians, etc., but the manner in which we chose those to fill the different quote would be a matter of judgement ... it would be haphazard.

Another rather academic disguise of a haphazard medical sample is a matched sample. This is particularly so in medical surveys - the case control study is an example. The haphazardly *matched sample* is commonplace in medical practice. A patient with a disease is matched according to different factors such as sex, age, race and social class with another person. Unless lists are available of all possible mates and they are then chosen as in a raffle-(an orgy!), matched samples are not randomly chosen and so no measure of reliability is available. Nevertheless, matched samples often successfully remove some of the effects of inherent variation between people. Patients are normally matched in pairs. If the matching is unsuccessful in that in fact each member is not more like his partner than those included elsewhere in the survey, this sampling method decreases rather than increases the sensitivity. Moreover, if one of the factors used in matching is directly and unsuspectingly related to the topic under comparison an existing association between a factor and the disease may go undetected. For example, cancer of the oesophagus is commoner in Africans born in Malawi than in Zambia, but this would not be discovered if a researcher had matched every Malawi African with the disease with a fellow from the same country. It is my view that medical research workers allow their match-making tendencies to run riot. Patients (when being used statistically) should never be matched as to race, age, social class or - would you believe - sex, without considerable mind searching. After all, who wants to be matched haphazardly? Although ... and why not? A change is as good as a rest. Nevertheless, if each member is not more like his mate than he is like the rest, this effectively decreases the size of the sample without decreasing the variation factor. Moreover, there may be a hold up in waiting for a good match.

A haphazard sample is therefore one in which the question asked is, 'Who will volunteer?' and answered subjectively by the research worker, 'You, You, and You'. It is often worse than completely enumerating a small population; for example, all the patients in a given hospital over a given period of time.

As with the survey into the rate of twin births in a central hospital in the middle of Africa there are many who will misinterpret what you have written and presume that your survey population is a *relevant population* in the field of study!

If in practice it is only possible to use a haphazard sampling method this should be made clear, because despite the lack of statistical foundations the work is still possibly of value. It could well serve as a pilot scheme or as a stimulus to others who have better research resources.

In summary therefore non random samples may be convenient to choose in practice but what is gained on the swings of convenience is lost on the roundabouts of reliability. Non random samples are liable to bias.

This subject cannot be dropped without mention of *Berkson's Fallacy - the case of the differing hospital admission rates.*

Although everybody knows that hospital admissions are not a true reflection of the general population, doctors still base clinical conclusions on them as though they are unbiased. In clinical medicine hospital admissions arising from a particular disease constitute a very haphazard sample of the population suffering from that disease. For a number of years some surgeons removed the gall bladder as a contribution to the treatment of diabetes, owing to an apparent association *in the hospital* between this disease and cholecystitis. The bias was caused by differing independent hospital admission rates and was exposed by Dr Berkson at the Mayo Clinic over 30 years ago, in 1946. Yet some medical research workers still fall into this pit.

Imagine that in St. Lucifer's Hospital the admission rates are 90 per cent for cancer of the lung, 10 per cent for gonorrhoea, and 50 per cent for correction of squints and that these admission rates are independent. Consider that in the general population there are 200 cases of lung cancer, 500 cases of gonorrhoea and 20 per cent overall prevalence of squint. Moreover, assume that squinting is not in any way associated with either of the other conditions.

(a) This means that 100 of the 500 gonorrhoea cases also squint. Of these 100 cases we would admit 55 (10 or 10 per cent on account of their gonorrhoea and 50 per cent of the other 90, i.e. 45, due to their squint). We could insert these 55 cases of squinting gonorrhoea in Table 2 which is based on hospital admissions. The table is completed by using the stated facts and applying the same reasoning, i.e.

(b) *Consider those with cancer of the lung who don't squint*
There are 160 such people and 90 per cent of them = 144 are admitted.

(c) of the 40 cases of *cancer of the lung who squint* 90 per cent of them =

36 are admitted because they have cancer and of the other 4, 50 per cent = 2 are admitted, not because they have cancer but on account of their squint. Therefore 38 cases of cancer of the lung with squints are admitted.

(d) Consider those with *gonorrhoea who don't squint.* There are 400 such people and 10 per cent of them = 40 are admitted.

Notice that inside the hospital, even though outside there is no association, 58 per cent of cases of gonorrhoea squint compared with only 20 per cent of cancer of the lung. It is as though the high cancer of the lung admission rate has pushed squinters into gonorrhoea beds.

A significance test would show a highly statistically significant association (within the hospital) between squinting and gonorrhoea. Some would go one step further. Squinting causes gonorrhoea!

Table 2 Details of 277 patients in St. Lucifer's Hospital with Gonorrhoea or Cancer of the lung in relation to Squint.

	Gonorroea	Cancer of the Lung	Total
Squint	55	38	93
No Squint	40	144	184
Total	95	182	277

b) *How many guinea pigs?*

Sometimes two are better than an army ... at least they make less noise.

W.T. Eldridge

A question which the professional statistician is frequently asked is, 'How many cases should I investigate?'

The would-be medical statistician, that is, the professional man who wishes to do an investigation, is often more concerned with the quantity than with the quality of his sample; yet, it should really be the quality with which he should concern himself. 'It's not the size, its the efficiency that counts', as the actress reportedly said to the bishop!

The answers to the question 'How many?' is: enough to be reasonably certain of detecting a meaningful difference if one exists. An experienced clinician can usually, if forced into a corner, decide what difference he or she would recognise as being of practical importance. Then the exact number is only dependent of knowledge of the amount the response varies in the population and the random sampling method used. One of the purposes of the small trial or mini run, more academically called a pilot study, is to estimate the amount of the variation in the population. Only if we have this estimate and the difference which would be considered to be of practical importance can we go on to specify how many guinea pigs are required. In fact, one works out the relevant statistical recipes, which so far we have managed to avoid, knowing the practically important difference and the amount of variation. Next one calculates the sample size in order *to make* the difference significant in the statistical as well as in the practical sense. This is opposed to the more general use of the recipes in which we substitute the size of the sample, the variation factor, and the difference we have found, to see whether it is a statistically significant difference.

The usual situation, however, in medical research is that one has to resort to a 'guesstimate' of how many to investigate. Is the guess of a statistician better than your own? Should you be asking a statistician how many? Probably not, if you bear in mind the following points.

There is the story of the two male centipedes who were watching a pretty girl centipede going down the street, and the one said to the other, 'That's a nice pair of legs, pair of legs, pair of legs...' It is more reassuring, as well as more pleasant, if your research finding is apparent in many as opposed to a few. We all like big samples but there is nothing special about the number 100 - centipedes may disagree! Although not trying to underestimate the worth of large samples, the advances in the science of statistics have tended to decrease rather than to increase the samples sizes required. As medicine has progressed so has statistical theory and small numbers can be analysed powerfully.

The size of the sample reflects only the precision of the work and has nothing to do with the problem of whether the results are systematically off target or biased. Moreover, a sample of 100 is normally only twice as good, statistically, as one of 25, although there is four times the amount of work. That is because precision usually increases not in direct proportion to the sample size but in proportion to the square root of the sample size. Therefore, to take a sample which is twice as precise as the initial sample, four times as many subjects must usually be included. It stands to reason, of course, that to treble precision the size of the sample must be increased to nine times the original.

Two golfing terms are relevant while talking about sample size. Firstly, 'sudden death' on the golf course is where the competition ends after an unspecified number of holes have been played, depending on the scores as the play off progresses. Statistically, unless special precautions are taken, it is wrong to determine the sample size as the results become available. Unless care is taken to allow for this in the analysis this decision must be made before the project is started. The one notable exception is the group of sequential methods - the 'match play' type of approach associated in medical circles mainly with the name of Professor Peter Armitage.

Consider as an instance of sequential methods a clinical trial of two drugs where the patients are tested in pairs, one of each pair receiving on the basis of random allocation one only of the two alternative drugs. If the patient on Drug A shows a better effect Drug A 'wins the hole' and so on along the course. Limits are initially drawn and the trial ends immediately a boundary is reached. The drugs each have their own boundary and the drug reaching its boundary first wins, as it were, the clinical trial but the number of pairs of patients included is only decided as the trial ends (Figure 1).

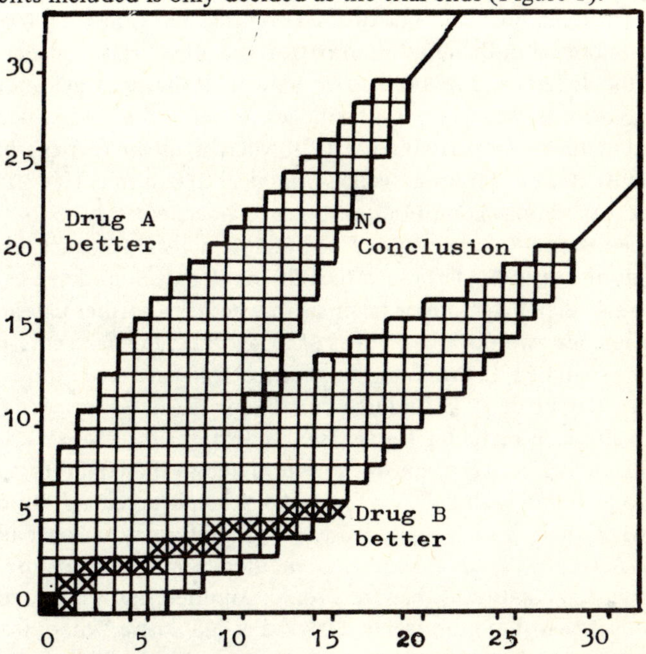

Fig. 1 An instance of sequential methods: A clinical trial of two drugs where the patients are tested in pairs.

How are the particular boundaries which are to be used determined? This depends not on the extent by which people vary but on the statistical manner in which they vary, and this must be decided beforehand. A decision beforehand must also be taken about (a) the size of the difference which if it existed would be of practical importance: (b) how convinced we want to be of a conclusion in favour of one of the drugs being real, and not due to chance, and (c) how determined we wish to be of getting a conclusive result in that particular trial. This last factor, statistically called the 'power', is essential because if there is no difference in the effectiveness of the drugs it would be possible to continue the trial for ever - neither drug boundary would be reached. We must therefore set a boundary to limit how far we are prepared to go (bishop speaking to the actress!).

Once the trial starts the results are usually drawn on a chart in which three boundaries are already in place; that for the conclusion that Drug A is better than B, that for B being better for A and that for no definite conclusion either way. With these boundaries on the chart one of the advantages of sequential methods is that no arithmetic is required. Some further good news is that if the information required from each pair of patients is only a decision, a vote, in favour of one of the two drugs the sequential trials are usually economical in the number of patients required. (Of course if the effect of the different drugs on the two patients is that they are undecided - unable to vote - then they are not included further in the trial.) Therefore sequential methods are particularly useful where a disease carries a bad prognosis because it is dangerous as well as unethical to continue giving inferior treatment for a serious condition for longer than is necessary.

Why, then, are they not always used? Because medical statistics, like life, is full of ifs and buts. We have seen that the results are considered as each pair votes and then a decision is taken as to whether a further pair are required. There are two obvious sources of delay. First the pairs entering the trial are matched. If the conditions for matching are made too complicated there may be delay in finding a suitable mate (actress speaking!). Therefore although matching for age, sex, severity of the disease, area of origin etc., etc., effectively removes variation due to these factors it is unsuitable to match in such detail in sequential trials. The second source of delay is when there is a long time lapse in waiting for a result once the people are matched (actress again!). Sequential methods are therefore more useful in acute medical conditions than in chronic. Another disadvantage of sequential methods is that the information analysed is qualitative, win or lose, and this can mean there is a loss of detail - not only of a quantitative nature but also in relation to the incidence of drug side effects.

Sequential methods are the most notable exception to the more general rule that the number of people to be studied should be determined before doing the project. It is also wise to use this number to estimate the precision before starting - particularly in the situation where available subjects are few. It may be decided that there is not sufficient material to start at all.

In general when quoting results, e.g., Drug A is significantly better than Drug B, the size of the sample has already been taken into account. We do not say, 'The difference is significant and moreover there is a very big sample', as though this adds more support. In fact, as we will see in a later chapter, only large differences are detected as statistically significant by small samples and in this sense if a difference is statistically significant and there is a very small sample, this implies the possibility of a big difference which is of presumably greater practical import.

Missing results

One of the problems with medical sample sizes not referable to golf is that of the *missing results.* Who ever heard of a golfer missing out a hole, particularly the nineteenth? Even though cases are omitted from the results, they should not be forgotten. The reason for their omission, whether it be due to failure to attend the clinic, or death, is important.

A drug firm ran a drug trial comparing two hypotensive agents on each of 100 patients. Thirty-seven improved more on Drug A; 14 on Drug B; and 30 were undecided. Do you agree that Drug A is better? It depends on the outcome of the test on the 19 patients gone missing. They might have dropped dead on Drug A or, of course, they might have felt so much better that they failed to keep up their clinic attendances. Missing results are one of the commonest and sneakiest ways of biasing results and to some extent missing results are more important than the others.

In surveys, particularly postal surveys, people also fail to respond. Sometimes as many as half the people receiving an invitation to participate in a medical survey by post will remain non responders. They constitute a considerable source of bias. In effect the problems are the same as a sample of volunteers - we are uncertain whether the factors motivating a person to reply are relevant to the subject of the investigation.

Of course results go missing, but let us at least be open about it. C.E. Ayres says, 'A little inaccuracy saves a world of explanation', and it is particularly enticing to fail to mention missing results. To me the thing to do is to be completely honest, state what has happened, what steps have been taken to try to trace the truants, and how likely you think they are to bias the results.

In the recent survey of journals, mentioned in the first chapter of this book, 28 doctors were dishonest in that they concluded their papers reporting on fewer cases than those with which they started out. They neither explained why these results took leave of absence nor did they apologise for this possible source of bias.

Remember that the sample size, if there are no missing results, only affects precision, not bias. To some extent a big biased sample is worse than a little biased sample, because it has taken more effort.

In conclusion

The best sample is one selected by a person fully conversant with the topic of the survey, the allocation of available resources and the principles of good sampling. What constitutes a good sample? One that is of sufficient size to be precise, sufficiently on target to be representative, and as convenient as possible both in methods of selecting those which are to be included and in administration so that those included can easily be reached for investigation. Often in medical research we are obliged to settle for a haphazard sample. My advice then is to use it, report it, but be aware of the pitfalls and, above all, to be honest about it.

7. How will the data be presented?

With signs and symptoms processed in computers
With patients' histories on punched-cards coded,
Old teaching ways ere long will be outmoded.
For philosophic profs, loquacious tutors,
Their classes' cool derision won't be spared
If they dilate on clinical impression
And quote no coefficients of regression,
Significance with t-test or chi-squared
Or standard deviations (i.e. sigma)
Mandatory now in scientific thinking -
Clinicians' aphorisms not hoodwinking
The unbelieving young; 'folk-lore' their stigma,
Technocracy ascends: it is our fate
Illiterate to be, but numberate.

Anon

This amusing sonnet was once surrepticiously slipped under my door. Of course there is much more to the practice of medicine that the scientific method. There is an art in detecting clinical signs, in giving a patient and relatives reassurance and the feeling that the doctors are capable; and we have already said that clinical impressions are usually the basis for putting statistics into operation.

There is also the need for basing medical decisions on as sound a mathematical footing as possible. To obtain results other than clinical impressions is one thing; to obtain meaningful results is quite another; to collate, summarise and present them in such a way that they are of real value poses further problems which we will now discuss.

Data on an individual

Problems arise as to how the data will look on an individual as well as on the whole sample. Now is the time to plan how the data on a subject will be recorded. For example, now is the time to check that a questionnaire, if you are driven to use one, is usable. The pilot study will assist.

Can the answers to coded? Remember too, that if the information is to be coded and put onto punch cards the necessary space must be allotted on the questionnaire itself or a separate transcription sheet designed. In either case, now is the time to discuss the format with the punch card operators, if the data are going onto cards.

Data on the sample

The presentation of the data on all the subjects may pose problems in practice as well as in theory. If you feel you could use the help of a professional statistician, why not go along and ask for it?

He or she can advise not only upon whether the findings can be meaningfully summarised but also whether the volume of work warrants the trouble of coding, transferring to punch cards, and sorting by a computer or other machine. For instance, I have often found it convenient to summarise data on individual cards and hand sort the cards or, if there are less than about 80 patients in the sample, to transfer the information to a large sheet of paper with one patient to a line so that all the information can be seen at once.

Should the volume of results warrant the use of a computer it is important to know at this planning stage that the facilities are available. This point must be cleared up before embarking on a project because the project must be tailored to the facilities. Self-evident, the reader might say. Would that this were true. But even if you are convinced that you do not need advice, remember 'to ask advice is to tout for flattery'. Of course I find it doesn't always work that way! Asking generally costs very little time or money - a failure to ask can prove expensive in both. Two words of warning about computers and statisticians. It is dangerous to hand your work over to a computer expert, or a statistician for that matter, who does not fully understand the background to the problem. *You* know that blood pressures and blood glucose are related, if not directly then indirectly, through obesity and through age. Does the statistician or the computer?

It is dangerous to allow computer experts and statisticians to analyse your data in such a way that you do not fully understand what has gone on. In fact, the statistician should spell out the analysis to the researcher's complete satisfaction and understanding or the researcher should not use it. It is possible that if you do not keep control over your data it will take over control of you!

Meanwhile it is as well to know that there are two kinds of statisticians - and I do not mean the obvious good/bad and male/female dichotomy. Both kinds are usually interested in you and your statistics but the difference (bishop speaking to actress!) is in where their priorities lie. The better kind use statistical principles to help you gain more insight into your data. Alas, the other kind seem to use your data so that it seems to be of secondary importance to their statistical ambitions.

Tables and figures

How will the data on the total sample look? This is the stage at which to outline the tables to be used for presenting all the information. This constitutes a check, apart from other things, that all the data which is being collected will, in fact, be used. Otherwise why collect it? In drug trials with complicated flow charts this is the time to study those charts in depth and peruse the various pathways. Are they really the alternatives which would be useful in practice?

To digress rather, one of the common mistakes identified in the journals that I studied was given the heading 'Faulty figures and tables'. Figure 2 shows how you can stretch a point by emphasising or exaggerating the scale. Remember that the purpose of including tables and figures in any survey is either to summarise essential information or to illustrate a point. They should save words in the text and must, of course, be honest. It has been said 'that the

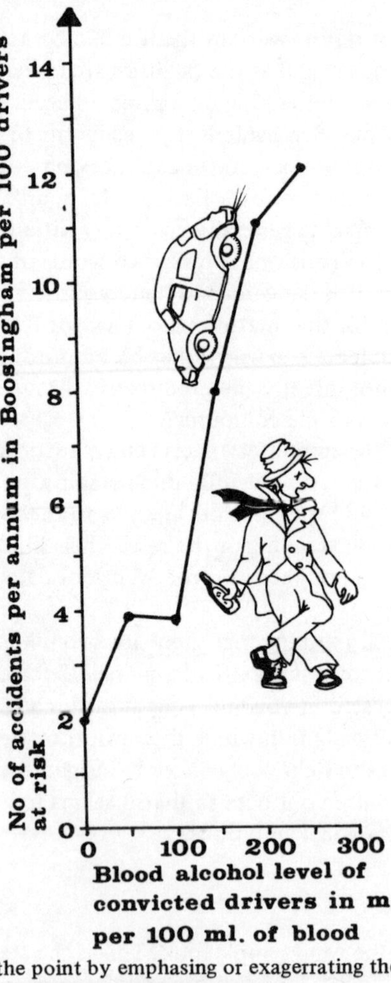

Fig. 2 Stretching the point by emphasing or exagerrating the scale.

reader deserves an honest opinion and whether he likes it or not he is going to get one'. Honesty is always the best policy, not least in the presentation of results. The scientific medical literature is not entirely free of the misleading nonsense used by those advertising branded pharmaceutical products. You have seen the 'before and after' type - a frown 'before' and a smile 'after' - not to mention the change of wardrobe, hairstyle and the bevy of exciting people of the opposite sex milling around in the 'after' scene.

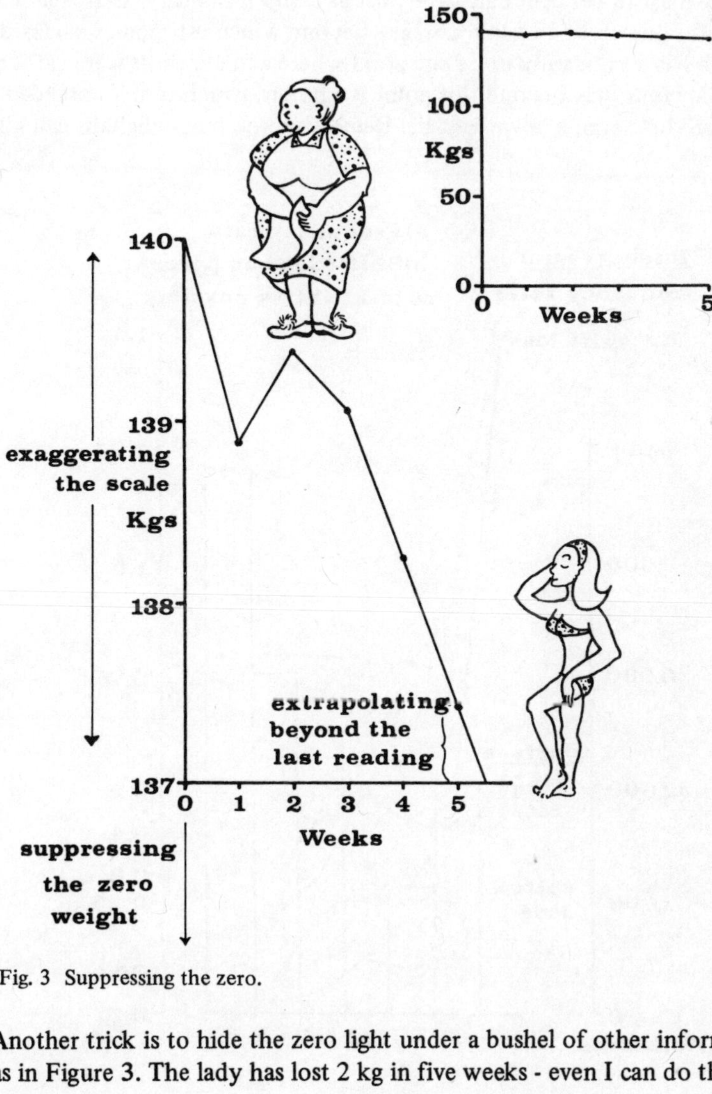

Fig. 3 Suppressing the zero.

Another trick is to hide the zero light under a bushel of other information, as in Figure 3. The lady has lost 2 kg in five weeks - even I can do that -

and part of the cheer in the diagram is provided not by the drinks which she has possibly done without but by the long stretch of vertical scale (all 137 kg of it) which she also discarded. This trick is called 'suppressing the zero' and it is effective when one wants less than 2 per cent weight loss to look like this week's news.

Figure 3 shows a third trick not connected with the axes but rather with the lines in the body of the figure. Where the line is extended beyond the information collected the trick is called extrapolation. In one article readers were shown a 120 per cent cure rate! Just as digitalis in heart failure has a recognised value up to a certain dosage - beyond which it becomes a hazard - so a graph has a value only up to the point where actual results were gathered. Pushing your luck beyond this point is a hazard which can, if extended too far, produce even a downright lie. Remember too much digitalis can kill the patient.

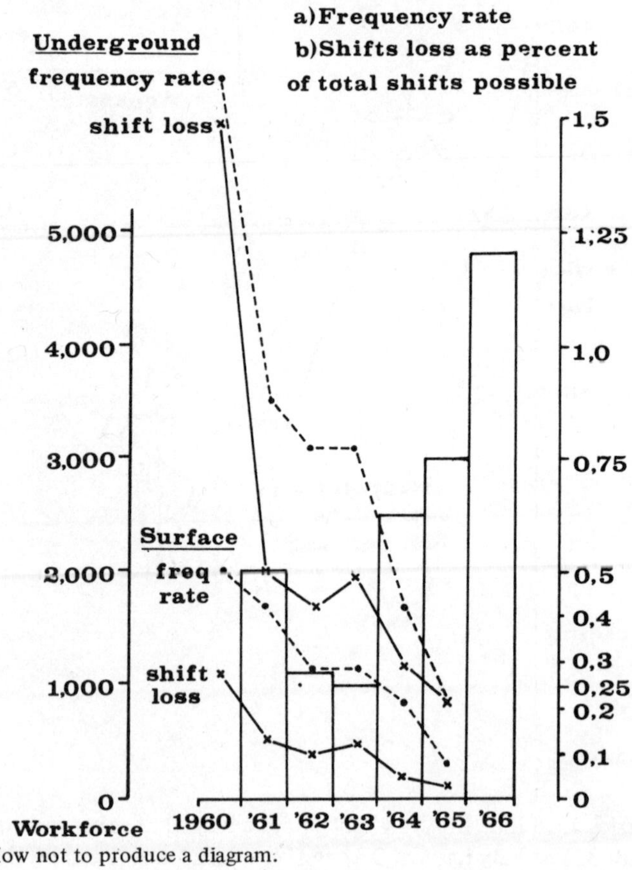

Fig. 4 How not to produce a diagram.

Diagrams and tables should not only be honest; they should be simple and an example of how not to produce a diagram is given in Figure 4. The figure is confusing. It has two vertical scales, and along the horizontal axis it would appear that one kind of information is reported from 1960 to 1965 (the lines) whereas other information is reported from 1961 to 1966 (the boxes). During the period of 1961 to 1965, in which time both lines and boxes abound, there is no relevant pattern and in fact the text does not appear to explain it further. Perhaps even the author got lost in the confusion and forgot what message the figure was meant to relay to the reader!

It is generally simpler to demonstrate one conclusion on each figure rather than many. If the information is counted, discrete or qualitative, like sex, as already described, it is normally enough to draw a pie diagram or a bar chart (Figure 5).

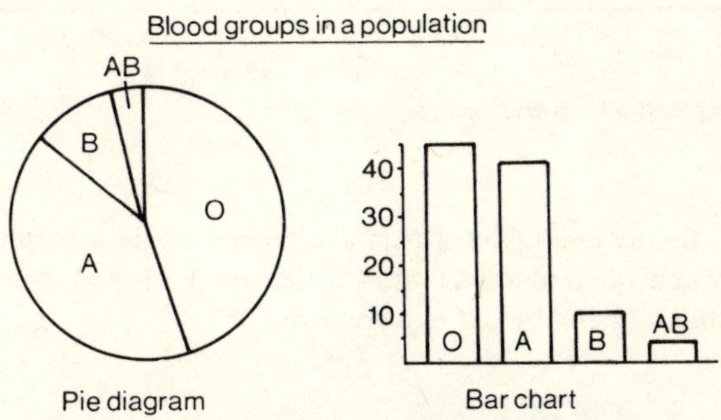

Fig. 5 It is generally simpler to demonstrate one conclusion on each figure rather than many. It is frequently enough to draw a pie diagram or a bar chart.

What if the information is a series of measurements or dates? The usual means of expression are histograms and frequency polygons. The measurements or dates are grouped and the frequency is noted. The size of the box reflects the number with measurements in that span in a histogram. In a frequency polygon (Figure 6) the middle points of the box lids are joined by straight lines before erasing the boxes. Usually the frequency polygon is continued onto the base line of the figure. This is not extrapolating as it is done only if the frequency in the adjacent boxes is known to be zero. The frequency polygons are generally used where one wants to represent more than one set of results on one figure as it is not possible to superimpose two histrograms and keep the diagram simple.

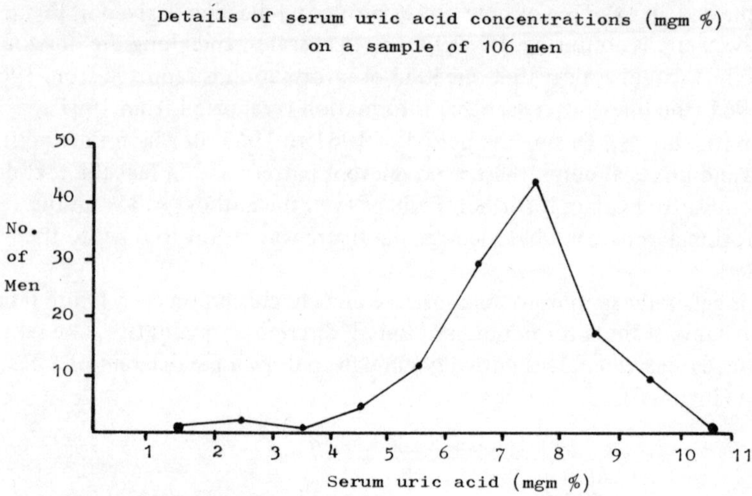

Fig. 6 An example of a frequency polygon.

In summary, figures and tables should aim to present data simply, honestly and effectively and when used in articles which are published they should save words in the text and be self explanatory.

Confusion can arise with histograms if the groups do not contain the same number of units of measurement. This is because the frequency in a group in a histogram must be represented by the area and not the height of a box. An example will help to illustrate the problem. Say with a new disease, Histogramosis, 10 patients are infants under 1 year, 12 are children aged 1, 13 aged 2, 10 aged 3, 8 aged 4 and 15 are aged between 5 and 9 years. Figure 7 is correct and Figure 8 is incorrect as it infers the highest prevalence is in the 5 to 9 year old group which, in fact, only averages 3 children for each year of age. Plotted correctly on the vertical scale in Figure 7 is the frequency of Histogramosis per year of age.

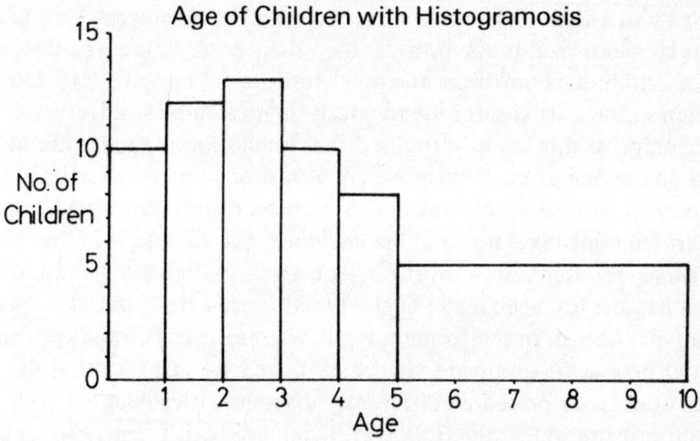

Fig. 7 The frequency in a group in a histogram must be represented by the area and not by the height of a box. This histogram is correct.

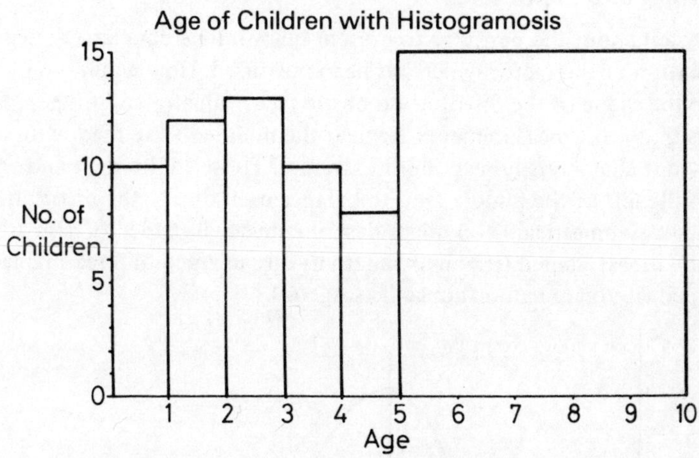

Fig. 8 This histogram is incorrect because it infers that the highest prevalence is in the 5 to 9-year-old group.

Presenting the data: the jargon

At this point I should like to draw the reader's attention to the jargon used in presenting results. Words such as 'the mean', 'the prevalence', 'the standard deviation' - what do they really signify?

The assumption - possibly hope would be a better word - is that the arithmetic in an article under review has been performed correctly. In fact, in the survey mentioned in the introductory chapter of 48 journals reviewed, I found 27 arithmetical mistakes and most authors did not give sufficient information in their articles for me to check their calculations. However, at the beginning of this book I promised that undue emphasis would not be placed on mathematics, so what we are now more concerned with is not the accuracy of the arithmetic but the correctness of the statistical terms. Quite apart from mistakes made in the *arithmetic* of the article in the journals surveyed; there was a disturbing looseness in the use of terminology.

Mention has already been made of the two different types of data - quantitative and qualitative. In the former people are measured (how sexy?) and in the latter people are grouped (which sex?). We have just seen that the two types of data are presented differently diagrammatically and it will come as no surprise to learn that they are summarised differently so far as the arithmetic is concerned. We have said that quantitative data, i.e. sizes, and measurements are more informative and should be recorded whenever they are available. Let us discuss their jargon.

Summarising quantitative data

The decision about the best way to present quantitative data largely depends on the nature of the factor which has been measured. How would you describe the shape of the distribution of the factor illustrated in Figure 9? It shows that most measurements are near the middle of the road, with a few way-out characters lying at both extremes. Those to the right and those to the left of the middle tend to balance each other - the distribution of results is symmetrical. You might describe it as bell shaped (if you are religious), breast shaped (if you are anatomically inclined or a sex maniac), or humped (if you are an orthopaedic surgeon).

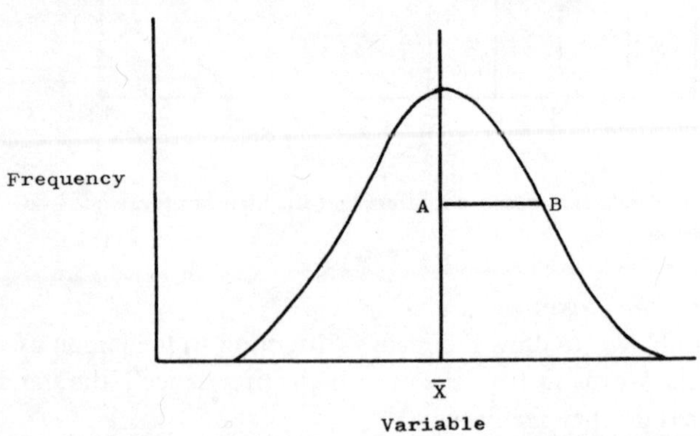

Fig. 9 Frequency distribution of a variable.

The Gaussian (Normal) distribution

To statisticians the curve in Figure 9 is a *bete noire* a black Arabian camel (which has one hump!). It is possibly true that many children these days look across the generation gap and see their mother as someone to whom, by and large, they owe their very existence and yet apart from this umbilical cord (and possibly the purse string!) there is little else to keep them together. Many statisticians look at that bell shaped, 'Gaussian'curve or 'normal' curve and see one to whom, by and large, they partly owe their very existence. Yet this curve divides statisticians into two classes. Possibly, as Oscar Wilde would have it, 'those who believe the incredible and those who do the impossible'.

The former are prepared to believe from time to time that the theoretical situation depicted in Figure 9 is not markedly dissimilar from what happens to the factor they are considering in practice - like a ghost, it is not really there, but they can imagine it is there. Are they naive? The other group pour scorn on this idea - like the duck's back, the normal curve for them holds no water. They don't believe in ghosts. The normal curve they correctly say occurs only in theory and is abnormal, unusual and in fact never occurs in practice. So far so good, but then this second group usually do one of two improbably things. Sometimes they transform their results so that they become more like a non-existent normal distribution and sometime they use so called non-parametric tests which say in effect that irrespective of the underlying distribution their answers are specific.

Female students might understand transformations more than their male counterparts who do not usually go in for expensive transformations of hair, eyes, etc. So disguised, females feel that they can handle life's situations better. All these artificialities reassuringly disappear in the bath leaving the dolly uncluttered and back in her original state. A statistical transformation is a way of tarting up data so that it appears different and usually more like a Gaussian or some other standard set of conditions.

Meanwhile the transformed data can be handled more satisfactorily. Such are the implications of disguise such as log and arcsin transformation and their more specifically pharmacological transformations, Probit and Logit. Fortunately at the end of the exercise we can do away with these numerical artificialities. The transformations have served their purpose and have helped us analyse the results but then we can reclaim our original data.

The question arises, how do we know when it is safe to assume that our factor is 'normally' distributed either before or after a transformation? There is special graph paper, probability paper, which has a peculiar vertical axis such that the effect of the hump in the middle and the tails at either side of the normal distribution are straightened. Plotting the data properly on this probability paper results in a straight line if the original information is in fact a Gaussian of 'normal' distribution. However, just as the distribution never exists in practice so the straight line on the probability paper never exists in practice and one is left with a better idea but no clear cut answer as to whether the line is too much off beat. One could use a formal test called a 'chisquared' test to decide about the goodness of fit to the normal distribution if one was determined to make a scientific decision, but by and large there are those that are and those that are not willing (actress speaking to the bishop!) to use the tests based on the normal distribution! The mean and the standard deviation are the tools of the trade for those who, like the actress, I suspect, are willing. 'In skating over thin ice, our safety is in our speed' so let us leave the 'normal' distribution for now and talk about the implications of the rest of the jargon.

The mean and the standard deviation

The *mean* is the average measurement (the value of $\overline{X}$ in Figure 9) whereas the *standard deviation* (the length of the line A B in Figure 9) is used to describe how far from $\overline{X}$ the other values X tend to be. To most doctors the *mean* or average and the *standard deviation* play innocent and prominent parts in medical journals - like virgins in a promiscuous society. They sit rather smugly together in print in their various disguises (such as $\overline{X}$ or M for the mean and s or σ for the standard deviation) knowing that they meet with the full approval of most editors of journals.

The mean and standard deviation serve different purposes but they are often presented together. Imagine a drunk in a casualty department walking along a straight line. The line lies at the middle of his (or her!) staggers and is like the mean in the middle of the results. The average amount the drunk deviates from his line is the standard deviation. They both hold a key to the diagnosis - too far from the mean as measured by the standard deviation - and you're in trouble. These characters give an article some tone and apart from their frightening appearance cause little trouble - or do they?

Some medical students show more animosity towards the standard deviation, the measure of variation, than they do towards the mean. They wonder why it helps the situation. The standard deviation shows us to what extent the results cluster around the mean and this is often important clinically, as well as statistically.

Serum creatinine levels in men have an average reading of about 9 mg/litre and serum acid phosphatase a mean of about 9 U/litre. Numerically the means are both 9 units but for serum creatinine the standard deviation is only 2 units whereas that for serum acid phosphatase is 4 units (Figure 10). Serum acid phosphatase is relatively more variable than serum creatinine.

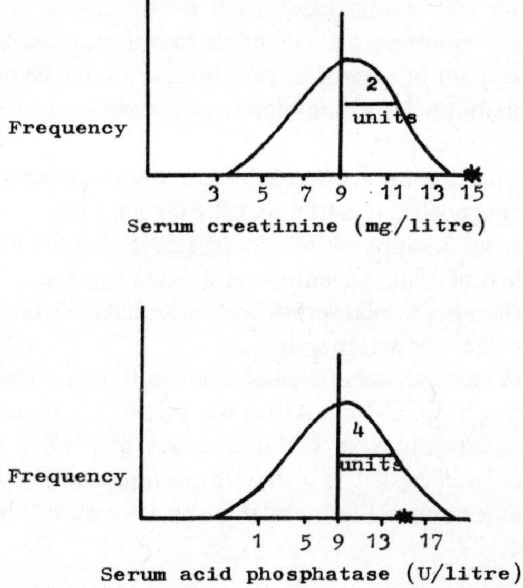

Fig. 10 Frequency distributions of serum creatinine (mg/litre) and serum acid phosphatase (U/litre).

Serum creatinine levels tend to be raised in patients with acromegaly whereas serum acid phosphatase is high in men with cancer of the prostate gland. Because of the difference in standard deviations an isolated result of 15 U/litre of serum acid phosphatase is less remarkable than a serum creatinine of 15 mg/litre. If the factor we are measuring (the variable) is approximately normally distributed (that ghost which haunts us!) 67 out of every 1000 healthy men have serum acid phosphatase levels as high as 15 U/litre but only 1 out of every 1000 healthy men have serum creatinine levels as high as 15 mg/litre. Laboratory results need to be interpreted in the light of the standard deviation as well as the mean.

Pathologists cut up dead people and I suppose we ought not be surprised that they tend to believe in ghosts. One can imagine a group of forensic pathologists at a conference:

> For God's sake let us sit upon the ground
> **And tell sad stories of the death of kings**
> How some have been deposed some slain in war
> Some haunted by the ghosts they have deposed.
> *Shakespeare:* Richard III

Pathologists seem to believe in the normal distribution and they usually quote upper and lower limits as well as mean values. The usual so called 'upper limit' is 2 standard deviations above the mean (13 units for serum creatinine and 17 units for serum acid phosphatase) and if we also believe in ghosts, the idea is that 2½ per cent of normal fit people have a value above the upper limit. Similarly 2½ per cent of normal fit people have a value below the lower limit (the mean minus 2 standard deviation): 5 per cent of people in all are beyond the statistical pale.

Remember, therefore, that these quoted limits are only markers, yardsticks - they are not diagnostic. It is true that the farther away a particular result lies from the mean in terms of the standard deviation the more likely it is to have a pathological undercurrent. A serum creatinine level of 15 units is more remarkable than is a similar serum acid phosphatase level - it is a stronger piece of evidence for acromegaly.

The converse is also true. A case of phaeochromocytoma referred to a major London teaching hospital from Africa was missed for about a year because the results statistically were 'within normal limits'. (The hospital was not of course St. Thomas's). The man with a serum acid phosphatase level of 15 U/litre has a result within normal limits. He may still have cancer of the prostate gland.

The variance

The value of the standard deviation multiplied by itself is called the variance.

The standard error

Sometimes the mean presents itself in print not with the standard deviation but with the standard error - in particular the standard error of the mean. One of the disguises of this fellow is $SE_{(\bar{X})}$.

The standard deviation and this standard error are related mathematically - it is quite easy to get from one to the other. The standard error numerically equals the standard deviation when it is divided by the square root of the number of results in the sample. Some may have thought the standard deviation and standard error were devices used to test alertness but they represent fundamentally different concepts.

We have seen how the standard deviation is used to measure the variation of primary data, for exampie, how pathology results vary in fit populations. The standard error of the mean is used to measure the variation not of the primary data but the means of samples. It is the standard deviation not of the primary data but of all possible sample means which would result if we repeatedly drew random samples of a particular sample size from a given population.

The standard error represents the inaccuracy due to sampling which we have already discussed as being inevitable because calculations in different samples give different values of the sample mean. In random samples the sample means cluster round the population mean but before mathematical conclusions can be drawn we need to know the extent by which all possible sample means are liable to vary. Only then can we hope to decide how to interpret observed differences between sample means.

Therefore the standard error of the mean measures the inaccuracy in drawing random samples from a population. This is why random samples are important statistically. The bigger the sample size the smaller the inaccuracy, and it is because the standard error is divided by the square root of the sample size that we previously commented that the precision in a sample normally increased in proportion to the square root of the sample size.

We have described how, in a population, if the variable approximates the normal distribution approximately 5 per cent of individual results fall above or below two standard deviations measured from the mean. The sample means are normally distributed if the random sample is large (this becomes so even if the variable is not distributed normally in the population, so long as the random sample is large) and so 5 per cent of sample means fall above or below two standard errors measured from the population mean. Therefore just as pathologists quote their so called 'normal limits' as ± 2 standard deviations from the mean, so statisticians quote their 'confidence limits' as ± 2 standard errors from their particular sample mean. In effect what they are saying is that in large random samples they are 95 per cent confident, that the true population mean lies within this 'confidence interval' (two standard errors in either direction of their particular sample mean.) It is a good idea to present confidence limits along with a particular sample mean as an indication of its reliability.

Mode

Before moving on to a discussion of the median, range, and percentiles - which calculated after the results are ranked, are some of the tools of the trade for those favouring nonparametric statistical tests - a word about the mode. It is another measure of the middle but uses least information and like 'the goodly apple rotten at the heart' it is the least useful. As its name implies it is the fashionable result in the sense it has the largest following - it is the value where the peak of the distribution lies. In the normal distribution it is in the same place as the mean. Sometimes in medical research one comes upon a distribution with two humps or two modes. (Figure 11) This is a useful sign that two groups of dissimilar people are mixed together - a statistical orgy.

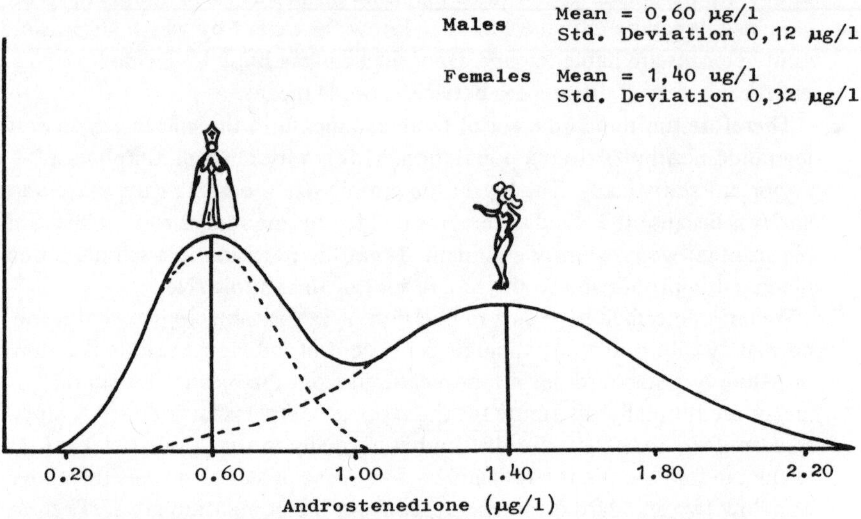

Fig. 11 Distribution of plasma androstenedione (µg/l) concentrations in a population.

The median, range and percentile

I admit that I have made rather a fuss about the so called 'normal' distribution - particularly as in practice it does not exist. This is partly because I had my knuckles rapped by statisticians reviewing my earlier book *Statistics in Small Doses* when I seemed to them to be too eager to believe in the normal distribution. Shelley wrote: 'While yet a boy I sought for ghosts'.

The median, range and percentiles are useful for those mature people who prefer to bury this particular statistical ghost!

The median, range and percentile are all easy to calculate once the results are 'arrayed' or ranked in order. The following results are not arrayed: 113, 118, 143, 126, 119, 96, 114, 103, 139, 116. Suppose they represent ten values of I.Q. which now are ranked in order or written in an array: 96, 103, 113, 114, 116, 118, 119, 126, 139, 143. Which is the *median*? It is the middle result - in the case of an even number of results such as the ten here - it is the average of the middle two, 116 and 118. The median is 117. Fifty per cent of results lie below the median and another name for the median is the 50th percentile. What is the *range* of our results? 143 minus 96 = 47. The range is the measure of variation often quoted with the median.

The mean and the standard deviation have the advantage over the median and the range that they use all the detailed information in their calculation in that if the second lowest of our ten I.Q.s was changed from 103 to 115, for example, neither the median nor the range would be altered but the mean and standard deviation would.

The median and the range can be usefully employed in statistical significance tests whatever the shape of the underlying data. Even if the distribution is approximately normal the median and the range can be used in statistical significance tests. Numerically, if the sample size is large, say over 30, the range is then about 4 times larger than the standard deviation - but the standard deviation is more efficient in measuring the variation in the data. The relative efficiency depends crucially on the sample size. If the sample size is greater than about 50 the standard deviation is about twice as efficient as the range. That is to say that a measure of range based on about 200 results in the normal distribution is about as reliable as a standard deviation calculated from 100 results. Similar implications apply to percentiles, which are useful but not so efficient as the standard deviation. When the results are lined up in order of size, arrayed, 10 per cent of the results lies below the 10th percentile, 3 per cent below the 3rd percentile, and so on. Two and a half per cent lies below the 2½ percentile and 2½ per cent above the 97½ percentile. Therefore, just as in the normal distribution 95 per cent of results lies within two standard deviations of the mean, in all distributions 95 per cent of results lies between the 2½ and 97½ percentiles.

The commonest medical use for percentiles is in the assessment of a child's weight for sex and age. It is important to realise that 3 per cent of normal children of that sex and age by definition have weights below the 3 percentile and that a light child may be one of the healthily light children and need not be one that is 'failing to thrive'. The 3rd percentile, like all such statistical tools, is only a yardstick measuring where one is, statistically speaking, and does not tell you whether an underlying pathological condition exists.

Correlation and regression

Before moving on to talk about qualitative data, a word about correlation and regression and some of their relations. They often appear together and are sometimes confused. Both require for their calculation pairs of measurements on the same individual, e.g., height and weight but whereas *correlation* is a symmetrical measure of the strength of the association between the two factors, *regression* describes how one factor (in particular the mean of that factor) depends on the other.

Regression is a simpler concept but we will discuss correlation first, because if the factors are not associated (as determined by correlation) the problem of how one factor depends on the other (as would be determined by regression) falls away. When we have two measurements on each individual and we are interested in their inter-relationship, the basis of correlation and regression, we usually first depict the results on a scatter diagram. (Figure 12)

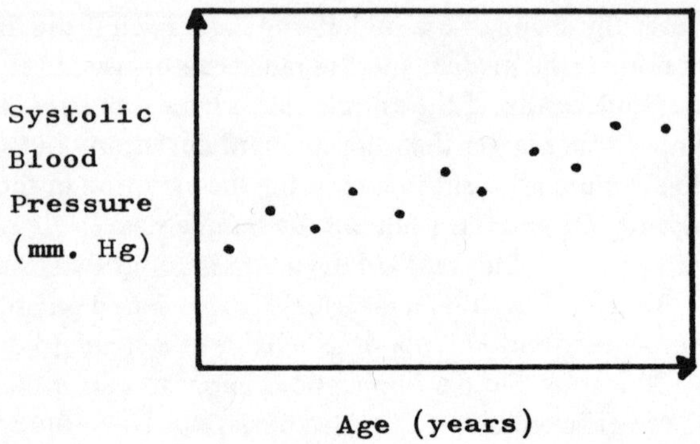

Fig. 12 A scatter diagram showing a relatively high correlation but low regression coefficient.

Correlation can be measured parametrically (usually given the symbol 'r' and called Pearsons Correlation Coefficient) by those who believe in ghosts, or non parametrically (usually given the symbol rho (ρ), and named after Spearman.) Either way it gives us a measure of how closely the two variables, height and weight, are associated - how close they are to the unlikely event of their lying on a straight line. If one increases as the other increases, as blood pressure does with age, then correlation is positive. (Figure 12) If one increases while the other decreases, like age and immunological response, correlation is negative. The maximum value a correlation coefficient can have in theory is one which signifies that the points lie exactly on a straight line. However large the correlation coefficient is, correlation only measures association, the variables are only 'good friends'. It does not mean that one factor causes the other. Height does not cause weight, tall people only tend to be heavier. I myself am overweight for my height but this does not mean I am underheight. The blame lies elsewhere: 'I am not hungry; but, thank goodness, I am greedy'.

Correlation, like disputed paternity, may indicate an association but it tells us nothing about the identity of the cause. Often the association is indirect through a third party. Blood pressure and cholesterol correlate but most likely indirectly through age (i.e., older people tend to have higher blood pressure and higher levels of blood cholesterol). If we wish to investigate the co-respondent, the third party, we can call in the private eye, in the statistical context, partial correlation. The partial correlation coefficient helps us to decide whether blood pressure and cholesterol correlate when the age factor is held constant.

When there is a sufficient degree of correlation to believe the results approximate to a straight line, it is the regression coefficient which is used to measure its slope. Regression tells us by how much weight tends to increase per cm. increase in height. The regression coefficient can be of any magnitude, therefore, and does not have a maximum value like a correlation coefficient of 1. Whereas correlation is used to measure how close is an association, regression can be used to predict the most likely weight for a particular height, for example. Regression coefficients and correlation coefficients have the same sign but correlation can for example be relatively high in that the points lie near to a straight line with a small regression slope, and vice versa (Figure 12).

In some medical research fields one is introduced to two other members of the regression family, ***multiple*** regression more commonly than *curvilinear* regression. What is the difference? One of my students cheerfully suggested that the curvilinear was female and multiple regression was male. Less cheerfully, curvilinear regression deals with the problem of predicting the most likely weight for a single particular variable - height, say - when the regression line is curved rather than straight. Multiple regression relates more than one independent explanatory or predictor variable, say obesity and age to the dependent or 'response' variable - say systolic blood pressure. pressure.

In multiple regression when a dependent variable is significantly affected by different predictor variables, it means the effect of each significant predictor variable is independent of the effect of the other predictor variables, i.e., it is present when the other predictor variables are held constant. For example, if obesity and age are both statistically significant in explaining the response of systolic blood pressure in a multiple regression analysis, obesity and age have an effect independent of each other. The partial regression coefficients are used to describe the magnitude of the effect of obesity and age on systolic blood pressure. By standardising the different predictor variables to the same mean and standard deviation the partial regression coefficients then reflect the relative importance of the effect of the different explanatory variables on the one response or dependent variable.

I think we are getting rather involved (bishop speaking!). Let us go back to the beginning and chat about the implications of the jargon used in presenting grouped or qualitative data.

Summarising qualitative data

Sex is an example of a qualitative variable which divides people into groups: 3 groups - males, females and professors, it is said.

Ratio, proportion and percentage

Qualitative information is commonly presented as a ratio, a proportion or a percentage. These terms are innocent enough but they are often abused. Sometimes they are mistaken for each other, sometimes they are misused and sometimes we allow them to lead us astray. We read, for example, that 'the ***ratio*** of male to female is 90 per cent (instead of 9 : 1). Although terms are only conventional the wrong terminology was the eighth commonest category of mistakes in the survey of journals referred to previously, and here is a case in point - another example of disputed paternity.

Then again, the terms are misused. It is always wrong to state the results of experiments without stating the numbers involved. For example, 90 per cent of subjects of an investigation may in fact be male but this could represent nine men or nine thousand. The emphasis we place on the difference of 90 per cent male and 10 per cent female is dependent on the size of the groups. Perhaps 80 per cent of film stars interviewed do use 'Noxanit 44' shampoo, but is this 4 out of 5 or 8 000 out of 10 000? It makes a difference, particularly to the nits, if in fact the shampoo does what its name suggest it can do.

I read the other day that 'it was particularly interesting to see that as the proportion of dead eggs increased, the proportion of the others decreased'! Surprise, surprise! Like salary cheques, if the *proportion* of income tax rises, the *proportion* of earnings for spending *must* drop. The egg finding is inevitable and not 'particularly interesting' as quoted.

The next treachery occurs when proportions or percentages, say, are inadvertently used for comparative purposes, then they can lead us astray. Suppose that a gynaecologist notices in his wards that over a period of time the proportion of admitted cases of cancer of the body of the uterus relative to all cases of cancer of the uterus has increased. He wonders why, and decides to investigate his admitted cases of cancer of the body of the uterus in much greater depth. Is this right? Has the gynaecologist overlooked the fact that because he has diagnosed some cases of cancer of the cervix very early by employing Papanicolaou smears, he has decreased his number of hospital admissions with this diagnosis? Hence, because the proportion of admitted cervical cancer is decreasing the proportion of cancer of the body of the uterus is bound to increase from this cause alone. So he could probably think of a likely answer without requiring to study his cancer of the body of the uterus at all. An increase in any proportion may well be important, but the decrease in the other factor in the proportion is perhaps the more important finding.

Morbiditiy rate

Instead of using proportions for comparative purposes it is more reliable to use a *rate.* If the gynaecologist has noticed that the rate of cancer of the body of the uterus was increasing he would have been off on a sounder footing. By rate, of course, I mean

$$\frac{\textit{the number of cases of a particular condition}}{\textit{the total number of people at risk}}$$

This may seem a simple definition in theory but in practice there are difficulties. With the number on top, the numerator, there are the problems of defining the disease and then the problem of finding all the cases. There are also difficulties with supplying the number on the bottom, the denominator. Care has to be taken in defining 'people at risk', the population, as well as in counting them.

In advanced countries attention is turning away from mortality or death measures to measures of morbidity or illness. This knowledge is used in medical administration as well as in research. As Charles Dickens said, 'It concerns a man more to know the risk of 50 illnesses that may throw him than the possible date of the one death that surely must come'. One can visualise the difficulties in collecting morbidity statistics compared with mortality statistics. Even for mortality statistics death certificates as to the cause of death are notoriously unreliable. With morbidity statistics not only does one have the problem of those who are not ill and think they are, there is also the more difficult problem of those who do not think they are ill, but are.

The enquiry often becomes involved with people absent from work for health reasons, A clerk with gastroenteritis, for instance, may well be at work whereas a similarly afflicted express train driver has problems! Other factors may also be very relevant; for instance, what other colleagues are absent, or even how keen the person is on his or her job!

Incidence and prevalence rates

Morbidity rates can either be 'incidence' rates or 'prevalence' rates and these terms are often confused with each other. What is the difference? An incidence answers the question 'how often?' and only describes conditions where the beginning is reasonably clearly defined - measles, pregnancy, for example, the disease is an incident. The 'incidence' of pregnancy in, shall we say, 1979, in a given place is the number of females *becoming* pregnant in that year divided by all those at risk! The 'prevalence' of pregnancy in 1979 is the number of females pregnant during 1979 divided by all those at risk. It refers to the condition rather than the incident. It includes those people becoming pregnant in 1978 who deliver in 1979 which incidence rate does not. Prevalence rates answer the question 'how common?' rather than 'how often?' a condition occurs.

Prevalence rates can give the number of cases in existence at a moment in time or during a period of time. The former is called the 'point prevalence' and the latter the 'period prevalence'.

It is, of course, quite wrong to compare directly incidence in one survey with prevalence in another survey - even if the arithmetic is correct!

Crude and standardised mortality rates

Rates can be crude or standardised and crude rates in particular are wolves in sheep's clothing. Crude rates must not be used for comparisons. The *Pocket Oxford Dictionary* defines crude as 'lacking finish' but many people are not warned and include crude mortality rates quite happily among acceptable tools of the trade.

The crude mortality rate is one of the vital statistics in relation to the community, generally recognised, by medical students in particular, as being of less interest than vital statistics in relation to an individual. The crude mortality rate is one of the statistics used by medical administrators and community doctors to assess the health of an individual population in the same way as clinicians use temperature to assess the condition of an individual. You know his ilk. The Crude Mortality Rate of Nappy Rash in 1966 =

$$\frac{\text{The number of deaths in Nappyrash in 1966}}{\text{The total population of Nappyrash at mid year 1966}} \times 1\,000$$

So far so good. The problem arises when we want to consider why the Crude Mortality Rate in Elderlea, 24, 5, is over 3 times that of Nappyrash at 10, 5 per 1 000? Do women driver's predominate in Elderlea? Are the doctors in Nappyrash of higher calibre than those in Elderlea. The answer is shown in Table 3.

Notice that in every age group the death rate per 1 000 is higher in Nappyrash than in Elderlea but because the population in Nappyrash is young the crude rate is lower. The people in Nappyrash live there during their employment and then move out on retirement to be replaced by youngsters not yet contemplating a rest from their labours. They move, in fact, to places like Elderlea, with its old people's homes, where they live their lives to the full until called to take their place in their own individual Crude Mortality Rate. We can readily do without Crude Mortality Rates for comparisons.

Table 3 Crude* and age specific death rates in Elderlea and Nappyrash

Ages	ELDERLEA			NAPPYRASH		
	Population	No of Deaths	Age specific Death Rate per 1 000	Population	No of Deaths	Age Specific Death Rate per 1 000
0-14	50	0	0	200	1	5
15-29	200	1	5	500	3	6
30-44	250	1	4	800	6	7,5
45-59	600	5	8	400	4	10
60-74	600	24	40	80	4	50
75+	300	38	127	20	3	150
TOTAL	2000	69	34,5*	2000	21	10,5*

* Crude Death Rates: ... Elderlea 34,5 Nappyrash 10,5

We have already discussed the problem of making comparisons between samples of different ages in the section about control groups. Let us take this opportunity to look at two methods of standardising for age: the direct and the indirect methods.†

Direct standardisation

We have already mentioned the fact that in each age group in Nappyrash the death rate is lower than in Elderlea. One way of eliminating the effect of the two different age structures would be to calculate how many deaths would have occurred in Nappyrash if the population of Nappyrash had been in fact the same as Elderlea. For example, instead of 200 people under 15 there would have been 50. Therefore, instead of one death in 200 there would have been 0,25. Similarly, in the 15 - 29 age group, instead of three deaths out of 500 there would have been 1,20 in 200. Continuing to the bottom of the table there would have been over 84 deaths in Nappyrash had the population been that of Elderlea giving an Age Standardised Mortality Rate of 42 per 1 000. This is 20 per cent higher in Nappyrash than in Elderlea with which it is now directly comparable.

This method of allowing for the differences in ages in two populations is called *direct standardisation* and to use this method one applies different sets of age specific death rates to one population, that of Elderlea in the example. Sometimes one uses a standard population structure to which both sets of mortality experience are related to estimate the number of deaths that would have occurred in both places had their population been that of the standard population. The particular population group chosen is that considered to be most relevant and different answers result depending on the different

† You may prefer to proceed directly to Chapter 8 (page 70).

standard population need. Although the actual choice of standard is immaterial in that differences due to differences in age structure are removed the more accurate the population structure the more reflective of reality is the actual result.

Indirect standardisation

This is the method most frequently used when numbers are small and when the mortality of a number of different subgroups within a population is to be compared. It requires different basic information from that needed for direct standardisation, namely the age (and sex) distribution of the different subgroups, their total number of deaths plus the age (sex) specific death rates of some carefully chosen standard population. Remember for direct standardisation the age specific death rates were required in all the populations for comparison.

To standardise for age, using the indirect method, the standard age specific mortality rates are applied to each of the subgroups so that the 'expected' number of deaths becomes known in each age group. These can then be added to give the grand total of expected deaths. The ratio of the actual number of deaths observed to this total number of expected deaths can be converted into a standardised rate by multiplying it by the national (or standard) mortality rate. Particularly when comparing occupational mortality, it is simple and more revealing to use the simple ratio (or 100 times the ratio):

$$\frac{\text{Actual number observed}}{\text{Expected number}} \times 100$$

which is called the Standardised Mortality Ratio (S.M.R.). This standardised mortality ratio has been much used in exposing specific occupational hazards, particularly when individual diseases are examined. The high S.M.R. for hepatic cirrhoses shown by publicans is an often quoted example.

As an example of how indirect standardisation works, suppose we have a population of doctors and a population of dockers with the national age specific mortality rate from cancer of the lung as shown. (Table 4)

Table 4 Population of Doctors and Dockers and National Cause/Age Specific Death Rates.

Ages	Doctor Population	Docker Population	Cause Specific Death Rate from Cancer of the lung per 100 000
0-14	0	0	0
15-24	0	10 000	4
25-34	15 000	30 000	12
35-44	15 000	30 000	86
45-54	10 000	25 000	416
55-64	5 000	20 000	990
TOTAL	45 000	115 000	34

Suppose 53 doctors and 498 dockers were known to have died from cancer of the lung in a particular year.

One would have expected from the standard death rates 1,8 doctor deaths (age group 25-34) plus 12,9 (35-44) plus 41,6 (45-54) plus 49,5 (55-64) giving a total of 105,8. In other words, only half the doctors died that one might have expected from this cause, or put in statistical terms the S.M.R. equals 50 per cent for doctors.

For the dockers one would expect, using similar arithmetical methods, about 332 deaths, but as there were actually 495, the S.M.R. equals approximately 150 per cent for dockers.

Therefore doctors have fewer deaths than expected and dockers have more than expected. We have thus summarised our information allowing for the different age distributions. We could follow up this information by trying to identify different reasons for the high rate in dockers - more spare cash and more inclination to strike - the matches!

Research workers can use these standardisation methods in medical surveys when the groups being contrasted have markedly different age distributions. They can be adapted to standardise for different socio-economic groups, countries of origin, etc.

Cause and age/sex specific mortality rates (Table 5)

In standardising directly and indirectly for age we have met the cause specific mortality rate and the age specific mortality rate. The cause of death is based on what is written on the death certificate and is only as accurate as the medical profession makes it! Another pitfall is that the W.H.O. international classification of disease which is useful for classifying the cause of death, is revised from time to time so that comparisons over a long time period are difficult - even if one remembered to standardise for differences

Table 5 Table of a selection of mortality statistics

DEFINITIONS	COMMENTS
1. *Crude Death Rate* $= \frac{\text{No of deaths during year X}}{\text{mid year population}} \times 1\,000$	1. Depends on accurate death registrations for numerator 2. Depends on census for denominator 3. Not to be used for comparisons
2. *Age Specific Mortality Rate* $\frac{\text{No of deaths during year X of people aged Y}}{\text{mid year population of people aged Y}} \times 1\,000$	1. Basis of standardised mortality rates 2. Basis of life expectancy tables 3. Total picture = 'force of mortality'
3. *Cause Specific Mortality Rate* $\frac{\text{No of deaths during year X from cause Y}}{\text{mid year population}} \times 100\,000$	1. Depends on accurate death certification 2. Diseases defined Internationally by W.H.O. 3. Multiplied by 100 000 as numbers small
4. *Maternal Mortality Rate* $\frac{\text{No of maternal deaths associated with pregnancy during year X}}{\text{Total live and stillbirths year X}} \times 1\,000$	1. Usual denominator in a rate 'number at risk' not determinable 2. In developing countries stillbirths excluded from the denominator
5. *Stillbirth Rate* $\frac{\text{No of stillbirths year X}}{\text{Total live and stillbirths year X}} \times 1\,000$	1. A stillbirth is a delivery after 20 weeks gestation with a foetus never breathing or showing signs of life 2. Depends on accurate knowledge of the dates of commencement of pregnancy 3. In doubt a birth weight of over 500 g is accepted as viability.

6. *Infant Mortality Rate* $\frac{\text{No of deaths under 1 year in year X}}{\text{Total live births in year X}} \times 1\,000$	1. Considered the best index of health in the population 2. Lowest in upper social strata 3. Different denominator from the 0 - 1 age specific mortality rate (see definitions)
7. *Neonatal Mortality Rate* $\frac{\text{No of deaths (0 - 28 days) in year X}}{\text{Total live births in year X}} \times 1\,000$	1. Improved less than post neonatal rates this century 2. Large proportion of deaths associated with immaturity
8. *Post Neonatal Mortality Rate* $\frac{\text{No of deaths (29 days to 1 year) in year X}}{\text{Total live births in year X}} \times 1\,000$	1. Improved most this century largely due to improved survival rates from infectious diseases
9. *Perinatal Mortality Rate* $\frac{\text{No of stillbirths and deaths under 1 week in year X}}{\text{Total live and stillbirths in year X}} \times 1\,000$	1. Used because births shortly before and after birth often have similar causes

in the age structure with the lapse in time!

More reliable, and more useful are the *age specific mortality rates*, shown in Table 3, where the number of deaths in the numerator and the population at risk in the denominator are specifically limited to one age group. Age specific mortality rates are usually presented per 1 000 population whereas cause specific mortality rates are quoted per 100 000.

The age specific mortality rate is usually given separately for each sex as the age/sex specific mortality rates. Its usual disguise is q_x where q_x is the probability of people of age x dying in a given year. The age specific mortality rates q_x are calculated from the national death notifications (the numerator) and details from the census (the denominator). If q_x is plotted against x, the age, it shows the characteristic 'force of mortality'. (Figure 13). The risk of mortality is, of course, highest at the extremes of life. In the teens the sharp increase is due to the high accident rate. This drops again in the twenties before death due to other causes increase in importance forcing the rate upwards again. The risk of mortality is higher for males than females throughout life. Is this really because women wear men down?

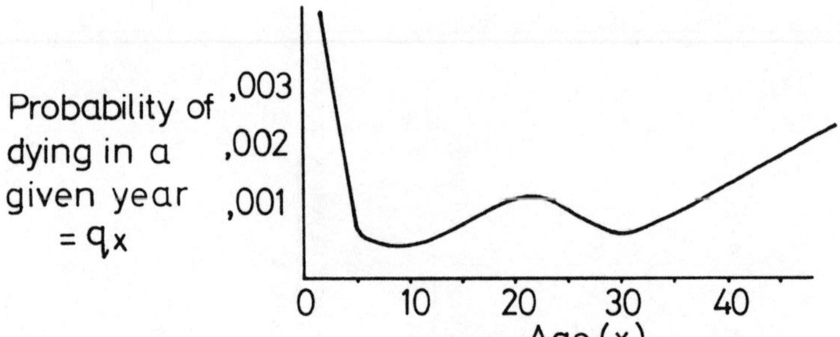

Fig. 13 The force of mortality.

Other mortality rates

Table 5 summarises the definitions and some of the interesting implications of some other mortality rates which are quoted by medical administrators. Politicians seem to get more excited about these vital statistics than do the medical profession. The cynic may say that anything quoted by politicians must be suspect and this is certainly true of figures used to summarise community health data. If one is not careful in *practice* 'damned lies' is a very relevant description. In *theory* they are relatively straightforward.

Life expectancy tables

For me, Life Expectancy Tables are a jollier more interesting way of presenting age specific mortality figures.

The construction of Life Expectancy Tables can be best understood by comparing it to a steeplechase. Look at Table 6.

Table 6 Life expectancy table constructed on the basis of a ficticious steeple chase (see text).

Fence (x)	p_x	q_x	l_x	d_x	e_x
0	5/6	1/6	12	2	6,42
1	1	0	10	0	6,70
2	9/10	1/10	10	1	5,70
3	1	0	9	0	5,33
4	8/9	1/9	9	1	4,33
5	1	0	8	0	3,88
6	3/4	1/4	8	2	2,88
7	5/6	1/6	6	1	2,83
8	1	0	5	0	2,40
9	4/5	1/5	5	1	1,40
10	3/4	1/4	4	1	0,75
(11)	0	1	3	3	0

The starting post is equivalent to fence 0 and two of the twelve starters refuse to start. The remaining ten horses all jump the first fence and one falls at the second. The nine remaining horses jump the third fence and one falls at the next, etc. Finally, three horses finish.

x = the fence reached
l_x = the number reaching xth fence
d_x = the number of l_x who fail to reach the next fence
p_x = the probability of surviving to the next fence having reached the xth
q_x = the probability of not surviving to the next fence having reached the xth
e_x = the average number of further fences reached by the l_x at the xth fence.

To understand the calculation of e_x consider the finishing post as the 11th fence. The three horses reaching the finishing post effectively go no further, and so their further run after this point equals zero. At the 10th fence four horses arrive, of which one succumbs and three go one further, i.e. $\frac{3 \text{ fences}}{4 \text{ horses}}$ = 0,75. At the ninth, five horses arrive one succumbs, one reached the next hurdle and three two more. Hence e_x equals:

$$\frac{(1 \times 1) + (3 \times 2) \text{ hurdles}}{5 \text{ horses}} = \frac{7}{5} = 1{,}40 \text{ etc.}$$

There is one interesting point illustrated in this steeplechase - the expectancy at the start (6,42 length) is less than that at the first fence (6,70 length). This means that those horses reaching the first fence have better prospects than all the horses at the start. This is due to the high drop-out rate before the first fence (2 out of 12). This effect has been deliberately contrived in this steeplechase but is precisely the same as in the case of life expectancy in human beings because of the relatively high infant mortality rate.

Nationally derived life expectancy tables usually have two extra columns, L_x and T_x. To understand these, consider the ficticious life expectancy table for hens shown in Table 7. All the numbers in the table are derived from the 5 values of q_x (the age specific mortality rates) and an arbitrary number of chickens being born (1 000 in this example).

The top line of Table 7 tells us that if the probability of death (q) for a live-born chicken before its first birthday is 0,1 (i.e. its probability of survival (p) = 0,9) out of 1 000 live born chickens, 100 will die (d). The number L, is the number of years of life lived by those 1 000 chickens that year, i.e. *before* their 1st firthday. (The mathematical assumption used is that those dying that year die regularly over the period so that on average they live 1/2 year each.)

On the top line the 950 years, L, is derived by adding 900 years (for 900 chickens living a whole year) to 50 years (for 100 chickens living on average 1/2 year). The next column T is the sum of the L column up to and including in that year. Therefore T is the total life lived by 1 000 chickens from the time that year starts (1 949 years on the top line). As 1 000 chickens between them live a total of 1 949 years, their average life expectancy from birth is 1,949 years, i.e. (e_x).

Similarly, the second line of the table tells us that the probability of hens not reaching their 2nd birthday having reached their 1st is 0,5. Therefore out of the 900 hens surviving their 1st birthday 450 will die (d). So, out of 900 hens 450 will live a whole year that year and 450 will live on average 1/2 year, i.e. 225 years giving L = 675 years during that year. From their 1st birthday 900 hens live altogether a further 675 + 270 + 495 + 4,5 years (the sum of the L column); i.e. T = 999 years. Therefore at their 1st birthday their further average life expectancy $e_x = \frac{999}{900} = 1{,}11$ years. And so the table goes on.

Table 7 Ficticious life expectancy table for 1 000 hens

x	q_x	p_x	l_x	d_x	L_x	T_x	e_x
0	0,1*	0,9*	1000*	100	950	1949	1,95
1	0,5*	0,5	900	450	675	999	1,11
2	0,8*	0,2	450	360	270	324	0,72
3	0,9*	0,1	90	81	49,5	54	0,60
4	0,99*	0,01	9	9	4,5	4,5	0,05

* Basic data on which the whole calculation is based

x = age in years
q_x = the probability of dying age x
p_x = the probability of not dying aged x ($p_x = 1 - q_x$)
l_x = the number of hens reaching aged x
d_x = the number of hens reaching aged x but dying before their next birthday
L_x = the number of years lived by l_x hens after their xth birthday
T_x = the total number of years lived by l_x hens after their xth birthday
e_x = the average number of years lived by l_x hens after their xth birthday

Life expectancy in human beings is therefore calculated from the age/sex specific mortality rates of those dying during the period under review. Therefore, life expectancy is about death. Also your present life expectancy, read off from tables, is only valid if the force of mortality has not altered between the time the tables were constructed and now. In fact one's life expectancy describes the death rates of those of one's own age and older who died during the period on which the life tables are based. It is a sobering thought that the only time one's life expectancy really applies to oneself is the year one dies, and these tables are only published later.

Life expectancy tables are most commonly used in actuarial practice. The reader may not agree with me that expectancies are fun but one must agree that they are financial wizards. Some of the biggest buildings in most towns bear witness to their success. Life expectancy tables have their chief use for medical research workers when they are used to calculate 'age corrected' survival rates and the same methodology can be used to construct tables showing survival rates after a particular surgical procedure. Basically one wants to compare survival in one group with that expected in some suitable control group. A chest surgeon with a low 10 years survival rate for geriatric patients may be less concerned than if he had a similarly low survival rate in infants.

In overall conclusion, remember that in presenting data, even if the arithmetic involved is current. if the design is too complicated, if the mathematical assumptions are wrong, if the control group is wrong, if the medical techniques are wrong then the answer to our original question will be wrong.

8. Shall we be able to answer our original question?

> What we want is not young men with fire in their bellies, but men scientifically trained so that we old blimps don't get the answer wrong.
>
> *Lord Mountbatten*

If what has so far been said had been in the form of a sermon it would probably have had the following text: 'Plan well before taking a walk down the pathway, clinical hunch - hypothesis - experiment - conclusion'.

It is easy enough to plan, more-or-less successfully the stage between 'clinical hunch' to 'hypothesis'. The problem is chiefly to spell out the exact question which one is trying to answer.

We have also discussed ideas about planning the survey or experimental stage emphasising the criteria of measurement, the person measuring, sampling and collating results. In my view it is also not only desirable but necessary to think about the final stage of the journey - 'experiment' to 'conclusion' - *before* setting out on each research expedition. Ask yourself now whether the data you intend collecting will answer the question originally asked.

Many of the mistakes seen in the medical journals arise at the final stage - the point of drawing a 'conclusion'.

In my assessment of the journal articles, of the articles reviewed:

In 29 per cent the conclusions seemed perfectly valid;
In 64 per cent some revision could have made them so;
In 7 per cent as the work was tackled, valid conclusions were impossible.

How had the researchers gone wrong? In what ways can we drive ourselves into such a corner that we cannot answer our original question even assuming that the arithmetic is correct and putting aside, for the moment the problem of *mis*interpreting the answer.

In the journal survey (Table 1) the second most common category of mistakes was given the heading 'conclusions without the evidence'. Sometimes the design was inappropriate, sometimes the sample incorrect and sometimes the detail was insufficient.

As an aside sometimes in reading medical reports one finds oneself expected to accept the answer without any data being presented at all! A rather cunning example is when an author writes 'Elsewhere[5] we have reported that bla bla bla ...'. When one looks up the reference at the end of the chapter one can see the subtelty!

Inappropriate designs

A colleague once decided to test the reliability of his method for measuring serum iron levels. He did not seek advice beforehand but enthusiastically measured a single serum iron level on each of 100 adult female visitors to the hospital. By the time I became involved with his work it was to reassure him that his mean result 1,4 mg/litre and his standard deviation, 0,4 mg/litre had been calculated accurately.

This is an example of an inappropriate design because *one* measurement on each of the 100 women, which he had analysed, may be used to describe the distribution of serum iron in adult female hospital visitors perhaps, but it tells us nothing about the reliability of the method. To test the reliability of a laboratory proceedure one serum specimen from one individual must be estimated a number of times, not one serum specimen from a number of individuals measured once. It is the variation on the single specimen which is used to measure the reliability of the method.

Another example of an inappropriate design is when a researcher measures disease associations in hospital. Say, for example, that medical records of 1 000 patients with varicose veins were revised and evidence was found that 5 per cent had clearly specified indications of rheumatic heart disease. In contrast, among records of 1 000 patients with inguinal hernias only 0,2 per cent had evidence of rheumatic disease. Even though the researcher may assure us that the two groups of patients were comparable in terms of age and sex, and even though rheumatic heart disease may be found to be significantly associated with varicose veins in the statistically mathematical sense it is not possible to answer the question · are rheumatic heart disease and varicose veins associated? This is because the strength of such an association *within* the hospital is partly related to hospital admission rates for the three different clinical conditions. The inappropriateness of this design is the same as that pinpointed by Berkson and described earlier in this book (page 34). It is in fact an example of what has become known as Berkson's fallacy. Possible associations between 3 diseases must be sought *outside* the hospital. The use of a large sample does nothing to remedy the error.

Of course, immoral associations in the medical statistical sense are not confined to opportunities inside the hospital walls. Suppose a headmaster suspects that poor performance at school is caused by a particular parasite infection. He arranges for his scholars to be given scholastic ability tests and to be tested at about the same time for the particular parasite infection. He might find that there is a highly significant association, mathematically, between the schoolwork and freedom from the parasite under investigation. This is an immoral association in that as yet we cannot determine whether the parasite is highly significant in the medical sense. It may be that those with the parasite coincidently have had few opportunities to perform well in scholastic tests - that these schoolchildren would be less likely to score high marks at school irrespective of whether or not they had the particular parasite living with them. A more appropriate design would have been to measure the school performance before some of the children became infected and to contrast scholastic progress of children who became infected with those of their classmates who remained free of the medical condition.

A retrospective approach is inappropriate in studies of personality in people who have had, for example, coronary artery disease. A control group does not compensate for the inappropriateness of this design. Not only is there the problem that heart attack survivors may be a biased sample in comparison with all people with heart attacks but there is the problem of personality change as a direct result of, as well as a risk of, coronary artery disease.

The incorrect sample

In my opinion no medical case notes are maintained with sufficiently meticlous care and attention to detail to make them reliable. Even in big teaching hospitals like St. Thomas's with extra junior medical staff and excellent medical record facilities the routine case notes are still probably a dead loss for most research purposes. Imagine you wanted to review disease X clinic records to see whether patients with disease X were overweight in comparison with the rest of the patients. What would one find? A certain proportion of records which had the information and some in which information about weight was missing. Mr Michelin Man, Sophie Tucker, me, Desperate Dan, Ten Ton Tessie, all the obviously fat people would prompt the doctor to record their weight. If the doctor was in a hurry, unless in private practice, those patients not particularly startling weight-wise would tend to slip through the clinic net, unweighed. The sample of records with the patient's weight would tend to refer to overweight patients - it would be incorrect.

Here is another example of an incorrect sample. I once read that in a trial to compare two dietary regimes A and B, 120 normal and 25 underweight children were chosen randomly and weighed clothed. For a six month period the underweight children were fed on dietary regime A and were given an antibiotic daily. The normal children were fed on dietary regime B.

What a mess! Not only was the sample *incorrect* but the treatment of one incorrect sample with the antibiotic added a further insult to that particular statistical injury. There are other snags.

The clothes add an air of imprecision and the imbalance between the numbers in the groups can be handled but is not ideal. How honest are children as far as diets are concerned? Were they locked up or otherwise prevented from obtaining extra food? If they were, did they not swop diets for a change? It is almost an insult to the random sample to mention it in the same context as this type of research - but it was published in a responsible medical journal.

This whole exercise is in the same class as not only reporting that the death rate in Birmingham is lower than in Bournemouth but that therefore a person living in Bournemouth is more likely to survive if he moves to Birmingham. You smile? Fine, but just keep your eyes open when reading the medical journals and your ears open when sitting in the doctors' common room!

The obituary columns of the last five years in one country's *Medical Journal* say, revealed that the average age at death of registered immunologists was 60,2 years compared with 73,3 years for surgeons. This difference in means may be statistically significant but this does not necessarily lend support to the argument that immunology is a dangerous life-shortening speciality! It is necessary first to check the age distribution of all registered immunologiests and surgeons to make sure that the relatively new speciality of immunology is not short of elderly fathers. If so, it is necessary to use one of those natty standardisation-for-age gimmicks before drawing conclusions.

This argument reminds me of Jean Paul Sartre's comment, 'When they wished to justify their actions they repeatedly gave reasons which were so dull they could not fail to be true'.

Insufficient detail

The proportion of cases of tuberculosis, $\frac{\text{TB admissions}}{\text{all admissions}}$, in the Lady Chatterley hospital has fallen significantly over the last quinquennium. So much so that the Secretary for Health is considering cutting down on his TB expenditure. Here is an example of shoddy thinking (not to mention the imprecise use of the word 'significantly') because in fact the actual numbers of cases of TB may have increased over the last quinquennium. In order to assist the Secretary for Health in arriving at a correct answer we need to remember the denominator and calculate the TB *rate* by dividing by the number at risk in the general population outside the hospital.

Similarly you could point to the hazards of clear weather as opposed to foggy weather in driving. More accidents occur in clear weather than in foggy weather because more people drive then. More people are killed on the roads by sober drivers than by drunken drivers, therefore driving while sober is dangerous. Nonsense. Yet this type of reasoning is all too common. The problem is that the denominators, the total number of sober drivers and the total number of drunken drivers, are missing.

The case of the 'missing denominators' can be given a more academic air. In a university teaching hospital, over a certain period, consecutive gynaecological admissions were tested for monilial infection. Out of 122 cases found with moniliasis, 31 were under 45 years of age and 91 were over. This led the author to conclude that monilial infection is more common in menopausal and post-menopausal women than in women of child-bearing age. In fact we cannot know in which age group, even within the hospital monilia is more common until we are told about the total number of gynaecological patients admitted in each group. Even then, of course, we know nothing about the distribution of the condition outside the hospital.

Whenever you read that 60 per cent of cases of a disease are one type of person and 40 per cent are another, ask yourself about the situation in the population, the denominator. Are 60 per cent of all the people one type of person and 40 per cent the other?

Another example of insufficient detail is when results go missing. There is the almost inevitable problem of subjects who are lost during the period under review. Worse than this is the problem of data which is actively eliminated rather than accidentally lost.

One of my acquaintances, a female sociologist, once studied people living in a sample of 100 houses. Using quite a rigid definition she classified the occupants socioeconomically into one of 4 groups on the basis of the nature of their house. She must have had much faith (she was a nun as well as a sociologist), great trust in her feminine intuition, or a deal of determination to prove her point because she then selected one typical representative of each type and failed to report on the rest. Even in medicine we are not usually so blatant as this - but you can sometimes see details about one 'typical' patient.

I suppose at this stage I ought to be completely honest myself and suggest folk do as I say rather than as I do. To some extent all women are liars. While highlighting many of the ways to cheat effectively I must admit I know others, but then no cheat worth her salt would discuss all her ploys in public. William Shakespeare said, 'What is a lie? 'Tis but the truth in masquerade'.

Sometimes it is not the total of results which is missing but the range. 'Remember that the man with his head in the fridge and his feet in the oven is comfortably warm - on average!' It could happen that a developing country might receive a flood of new immigrants and figures might show, correctly, that the statistically average family consists of 3,1 persons. Translated into housing terms this means 3 or 4 persons, which in turn means 2 bedrooms. But a builder would be making a big mistake if on the evidence of these figures, he built all with 2 bedrooms. For a family of this size, average though it is statistically, actually makes up a minority of all families even in a large sample. The majority would be larger or smaller. Probably about 40 per cent would consist of one person or two persons and 20 per cent would have more than 4 - in reality probably no more than 40 per cent would consist of 3 or 4 persons.

Similarly, in 'family planning' studies more detail is required than the average family size. Often in medical research, although the mean and the median are very relevant, the upper levels recorded on well people are important, particularly if it is your blood that is under discussion! It is often necessary to think and talk in terms of the distribution of results.

There is another example of missing detail which is a rather more subtle medical omission - measures of specificity while talking about sensitivity of a new test. In Africa there may be a test which is very sensitive for detecting albinos. It detects every one - it is 100 per cent sensitive! However, does it exclude white-skinned folk living on the African continent? Is it specific for albinos? Similarly one reads of new diagnostic tests which are very sensitive in that 99 per cent of people with disease X are identified. The missing data is the number of people without disease X who are also positive to the diagnostic test. If 90 per cent of these are included you are losing on the roundabout of specificity whatever sensitivity you gain on the swings.

Before going on to chat in the next chapter about the implications in interpreting the answer when a significance test is used, let us consider briefly three other common categories of mistakes pinpointed in Table 1.

The first is the case of the missing significance tests, when 'a significance test was indicated but not performed'. In one paper the author debated why among neonates with a certain disease the prevalence of one particular organism was higher in premature than full term infants. The prevalence was 8 out of 15 prems as against 8 out of 22 full term infants and a significance test would have shown that this difference was very likely only due to chance. The author was therefore rather premature himself in launching forth into discussing the whys and wherefores.

I heard a visiting Professor of Surgery, who now fortunately has become a University Vice Chancellor, telling the medical students that a 'recurrance rate of 1 out of 39 was obviously inferior to nil out of 52'.

I suspect that this error is made to a large extent by doctors not taught how to apply a suitable test and without easy access to anyone in a position to help them. This is probably why such imprecise sentences appear as, 'There is a slight dose response difference', 'The distributions are noticeably different'.

On 28 occasions the authors of journal articles claimed that they had in fact performed the necessary numerical gymnastics involved in significance testing and had achieved significant differences. My criticism here is that the name of the actual test used and/or the degree of significance attained were missing. This category is called 'failure to quote significance tests or significance levels'.

Serious readers, perhaps those reading articles while in the process of writing their own theses, need to assess others' results. In nearly every article that I read the biochemical and physiological methodology was described at great length but the statistical test used, requiring often only three to four words, was omitted. Just as there are reliable and unreliable biochemical tests there are good and bad statistical methods in different situations. We cannot automatically assume that the tests used where the name was not given were in fact correctly used. On the contrary, in 24 further cases where the particular significance test used was stated, it was inappropriate. For example, the samples were matched one for one, and no cognizance was taken of this fact in the analysis. I think it is important that the statistical test used should be named.

I also think it is time I dismounted and stopped riding one of my own favourite hobby horses. Most readers probably only want direction in assessing the statistical conclusions made by their colleagues. For example, what are the implications of $0{,}05 > p > 0{,}01$ seen in print?

Ref 5. Blacksheep et al. Unpublished.

9. Shall we be able to interpret the answer?

> In preparation for this coming generation much of great literature will have to be rewritten, else it will be incomprehensible.
>
> Always willing to be in the forefront of any new movement, I have made a start of Julius Caesar;
>
> Computers which have captured from the stars
> Their role of prophecy, discern a link
> 'Twixt body-weight and loyalty, such that p
> Is meaningful at less than point-nought-five.
> Thus would I rather have about me, men
> More to the right of distribution curves
> Than yonlean Cassius. He thinks too much.
> Statistic'ly such men are dangerous.
>
> *Lord Platt*

Firstly, a short story.

The bishop eventually married the actress. We next meet them in the waiting room of a genetic counselling clinic. As they sat together their particular problem was obvious. The bishop's domed head had clinical as well as clerical significance, his small face and short limbs were typical of those whom medical people term 'achondroplastic dwarfs'. The bishop and the actress had sensibly come to seek advice about the likelihood of their children, if they had any, also being achondroplastic dwarfs.

The bishop and the actress were advised by the genetic counselling panel not to have any children as each offspring would have an evens chance of being an achondroplastic dwarf. The bishop's wife in particular was upset by this news, so much so that she did not react to the chauvinistic comment to the effect that her husband was 'dominant'.

For a few years Bishop White accepted the medical advice philosophically but then Mrs White put pressure on her more sensible husband. Nevertheless the bishop adhered to the view that the counsellors' advice was correct.

Perhaps the actress persuaded the bishop that faith may adjust the odds in their favour because she eventually became pregnant. Their first child was an achondroplastic dwarf but he was such a happy dwarf that he gave his parents tremendous pleasure, and it was not long before Mrs White was the mother of a second son - another dwarf. This child was also little trouble, sleeping through the nights. The third son was remarkable in that not only was he a dwarf but he sneezed on arrival instead of crying. The fourth son was a bashful dwarf.

By this time the bishop was also rather bashful. *'I'm sure the medical estimate, that the odds are 50:50, is correct.,'* he said, *'but there is something uncanny in all these dwarfs we seem to be producing'.* It took more than 4 dwarfs to inhibit the ex-actress. She reassured her husband: *'It is obviously just bad luck',* she said, *'ignore it'.*

I am sad to recount that things went from bad to worse. The fifth child, yet another dwarf, was not very clever. The sixth child was a bad-tempered dwarf and by this time so was the bishop.

The bishop and his wife agreed that *even though there was no proof* that the quoted odds were incorrect, *for all the dwarfs could have arisen by chance* with the stated odds of 50 : 50, it was most suspicious. *'The line must be drawn somewhere'* said the bishop, 'if it happens again I will be sterilised'. (Doc-tored?!) It did happen again so the story of Mrs White and her sequential trial of 7 dwarfs ends.

I do not recount this story idly, but because some of the ideas brought out are pertinent to interpreting results from medical research and to drawing conclusions. The circumstances are fortunately different, but there are lessons to be learnt. Firstly, the bishop's wife's initial reaction was, 'It is obviously just bad luck ignore it'. This same attitude was held in the beginning by the bishop when he assumed the medical estimate was correct. This is akin to the English legal approach where in theory at least, a man is held to be innocent until shown to be guilty.

Statisticians also choose to assume that there is nothing suspicious going on at first. If a new analgesic is being tried we firstly assume that it is no better than its older competitors. It is up to the results to make us change our minds and unless the evidence in the data is sufficient we rather retain the view that any observed effect is due to chance alone. Statistically, this original viewpoint is called the 'Null Hypothesis', but this is a sophisticated way of saying to the medical research worker, 'I don't believe you until you convince me'. When in doubt, believe nought!. Of course a significance test is only concerned with what the results have established. Statisticians need not believe that all things not established by significance tests are non existent - they accept, though, that there is insufficient evidence to reject the Null Hypothesis.

The bishop and his wife hit the next statistical nail on the head.with their viewpoint that there could be 'no proof' ... 'for the results could always be due to chance'. I am often told that statistics never prove anything; that people vary, and any differences between their reactions could be caused by their inherent variability. If people were identical in their behaviour we could treat the outcome of trials simply. It is the fact that people do vary which reinforces the need for statistics, the subject developed especially to take into account this variability. Progress would be non-existent if our initial view is that we need convincing and our second view is that we cannot have proof and hence cannot be convinced. Statistical analysis produces a reasoned measure of doubt concerning our faith in the null hypothesis. Very rarely are juries given direct proof of a man's guilt, but it is their duty to sift through the evidence with an open mind to determine a man's guilt beyond reasonable doubt.

This reminds me of the verdict of the Irish jury. 'My Lord', said the foreman of the jury when giving his verdict, 'we find the man who stole the mare not guilty'. It is true that we cannot prove a new analgesic to be better, but with an open mind we can decide it is different beyond reasonable doubt. As Sam Goldwyn said, 'I am giving you a definite maybe'. Christopher Morley also underlined the point that we can never prove anything with statistics.

Con was a thorn to brother Pro
On Pro we often sucked him.
Whatever Pro would claim to know
Old Con would contradict him.

Be cynical of statistical principles if you wish, but people do vary and to produce a reliable set of odds with an open mind seems to me to be no mean achievement.

The final point made by the bishop is that 'the line must be drawn somewhere'. A measure of doubt, no matter how reliable, is a dead end if no conclusions can be drawn and no action taken. Therefore I disagree with Oscar Wilde when he said, 'The man who sees both sides of the question is a man who sees absolutely nothing at all'.

It is true that chance could always be the cause, but the time must come when the evidence is such that it is more realistic to acknowledge some other factor. Juries reach conclusions of 'guilty' and judges act accordingly. Statisticians prefer the innocence of the null hypothesis, but given sufficient evidence they will renounce it and accept that which the evidence proclaims. The line is drawn and it becomes reasonable to conclude that the new analgesic is really better.

In statistics it is essential that a line must be drawn somewhere and that it is drawn with an open mind. The line is called a 'significance level', and it becomes the yardstick against which decisions are made. The significance level is established before the results are analysed so that the conclusions are made as fairly as possible. Of course, you can look at the results and decide upon your verdict blindly. But as there are significance tests based on the laws of probability designed to guide one, it seems wiser to me to use them. It is difficult otherwise to be certain that your decision is not being influenced by some preconceived notion of your own or emotive language being used by the person quoting results. For example, some people hold views about numbers of female doctors. In a certain country, 85 out of 504 practicing doctors are female. Antagonism to female doctors by one writer is indicated by expressing this situation as 'less than 17 per cent of all practising doctors in that country are women'. This is true, but it is equally true that 'there is more than one female doctor in full-time practice for every five males'. This now infers that the female contribution to medicine is fairly substantial. The wording reflects the speaker's personal opinion and is likely to influence one's own thoughts on the subject. This is equally true with the results from medical research and it is necessary to measure the significance of the results, in such a way as to reduce the effect of opinion, preconceived ideas, emotive language or propaganda.

Originally, I likened the statistician's work to that of a course steward. Judging the results of races, by significance tests is only one of the aspects of medical statistician's work. Many punters at a race meeting have no conception of the preparation beforehand; they only see the actual race. Just as there is more than a lot of nags to a race, there are more than a lot of conclusions to a trial. Remember, a significance test is only as worthwhile as the preparation which has gone into collecting the data. Significance tests may support a theory, like a lamp post a drunken man, but it is the design of a clinical trial which provides the illumination.

Remember I made rather a song and dance about random samples - the samples where chance played a calculated part. The estimation of p depends on mathematical distributions, often χ^2 if the results are qualitative and 'Student's t' if the results are quantitative and approximately normally distributed. χ^2 and 't' describe what is likely to happen according to the laws of chance, i.e., they apply to random samples where chance determines who is included in a particular sample. When samples are taken haphazardly there is no mathematical equivalent known and so theoretically anyway we reach a dead end.

Let us apply the ideas so far in practice. Suppose we took a random sample of 100 English doctors and calculated their average I.Q. to be 120. Imagine in America the average I.Q. of doctors was 130. Applying the morals of our story we initially assume this difference is only due to chance. In fact, this could always be so, a difference which has a one in a million chance of turning up will turn up due to chance one in a million times. Nothing is impossible. Even if we decide the difference is statistically significant we could always be wrong about underlying reality. Nevertheless, we must draw some guide lines against which to measure the evidence. Such is the purpose of significance tests. The yardstick or significance levels commonly used are

0,05, 0,01 or 0,001 or probabilities of 1/20, 1/100 or 1/1 000. If we come to decide that the difference is statistically significant at 0,05 we are saying in effect that, believing that the results are only due to chance, as initially we must do, it is such a rare event that chance would cause such a difference in less than 1 time out of 20. An outsider has won. At the 0,001 level, chance would cause such a result only remotely - in less than one time out of 1 000.

This 'p' we see in journals, what is it? It is the probability of a difference as large or larger than that observed arising by chance alone; as such it gives a measure of the conformity of the data to the null hypothesis. The bigger 'p' the more the results are what would be expected with the null hypothesis true.

The smaller 'p' becomes - like a mini-skirt - the more willing we are to believe that a real difference exists. The smaller and smaller 'p', the more and more convinced we become that these results are not only due to chance; the more and more statistically significant the difference becomes.

So 'p' is calculated from our results using one of the many statistical recipes and we then compare it with our yardstick values 0,05, 0,01 and 0,001 which we chose to begin with. If 'p' is bigger than 0,05 we assume the difference is due to chance - the odds are so short that a favourite has come in, nothing significant has happened. As the odds lengthen and the outsiders with small 'p' turn up in our trials so the results become more and more statistically significant.

Assuming the American doctors' I.Q. on average was 130 and the sample of 100 English doctors' I.Q. was 120 a significant test could give the results $0{,}001 > p$. The conclusion would then be that American doctors were significantly more intelligent. Possible? 'Is anything impossible? Read the newspapers.' (Duke of Wellington).

As you see, everything in significance tests hinges on our calculations of 'p'. Three things affect it: the size of the difference between the different groups, the size of the variation and the size of the sample. Consider each in turn. Obviously if the average I.Q. in the English sample had been 125 instead of 120 the results would have been less significantly different. The bigger the difference between the groups the smaller 'p'.

The smaller the variation the smaller 'p'. This is because if things commonly vary a lot, a difference is not so remarkable as is a difference in a situation where variation is usually minimal. You are not surprised if a person who is emotionally labile, who is up in the air one minute and down in the depths another laughs. His moods vary a lot anyway. If a miserable person laughs it is more significant because his moods usually vary very little. It is because the smaller the variation is, the smaller 'p' is, all other things being equal, the emphasis is placed on cutting down on variation in sampling and experimentation. This way we are in a stronger position to convict the Null Hypothesis and accept a new theory.

Going back to the story of the achondroplastic dwarfs, it was only when more and more dwarfs were born that the bishop became really suspicious about the 50 : 50 odds quoted by the genetic counsillors. In fact, the larger the number of dwarfs the more suspicious he became; the smaller 'p'. If we look harder at the story of the dwarfs we can learn more about the relationship between 'p' and the sample size.

The probability of the 1st dwarf was said to be $^1/2$ or 50 : 50. That is to say that all things being equal in the long run the bishop should have had one dwarf every two children. Now the probability of the bishop and the actress producing dwarfs twice in a row is $^1/2 \times {}^1/2 = {}^1/4$ (the same probability as for you tossing heads twice in a row with a coin). The probability of it happening three times in a row is $^1/2 \times {}^1/2 \times {}^1/2 = {}^1/8$, four times $^1/2 \times {}^1/2 \times {}^1/2 \times {}^1/2 = {}^1/16$, etc. (Table 8).

Table 8 The probability of producing consecutive achondroplastic dwarfs with odds for each dwarf of 50 : 50.

The number of dwarfs in the family	Name of the dwarf in story	The probability of this number of consecutive dwarfs due to chance with the stated odds of 50 : 50
1	Happy	$^1/2$ = 0,5000
2	Sleepy	$^1/4$ = 0,2500
3	Sneezy	$^1/8$ = 0,1250
4	Bashful	$^1/16$ = 0,0625
←		→ 0,05 yardstick
5	Dopey	$^1/32$ = 0,0312
6	Grumpy	$^1/64$ = 0,0156
←		→ 0,01 yardstick
7	Doc	$^1/128$ = 0,0078
8	-	$^1/256$ = 0,0039
9		$^1/512$ = 0,0020
←		→ 0,001 yardstick
10	-	$^1/1024$ = 0,0010

Before the birth of Dopey, notice, 'p' was bigger than the yardstick value 0,05 and the results were not statistically significant. When the 5th dwarf

Dopey was born and Grumpy the results were significant at the 0,05 level, (i.e. $0{,}05 > p > 0{,}01$). On the birth of the seventh dwarf, Doc, the results became significant at the 0,01 level (i.e. $0{,}01 > p > 0{,}001$) and had the bishop and the actress had 10 dwarfs in a row and no normal children this would have meant $0{,}0001 > p$, which is very significant in the statistical sense as well as the medical sense.

We see that the larger the sample, with the same effects, the more significant the results become in the statistical sense. Even though initially 'we must believe in luck, for how else can we explain the success of those we don't like', gradually our opinions change and we reject the null hypothesis when we pass the significance level. Figure 14 illustrates the probability of the bishop and the actress, out of 7 offspring, having 7 dwarfs (the black area). It also shows the probability of them having other than 7 dwarfs out of 7 children. Producing dwarfs is really a sequential procedure and Figure 14 shows the probabilities of all possible outcomes with 7 children assuming, as we initially do, that the null hypothesis is true, i.e. that the odds for each are 50 : 50.

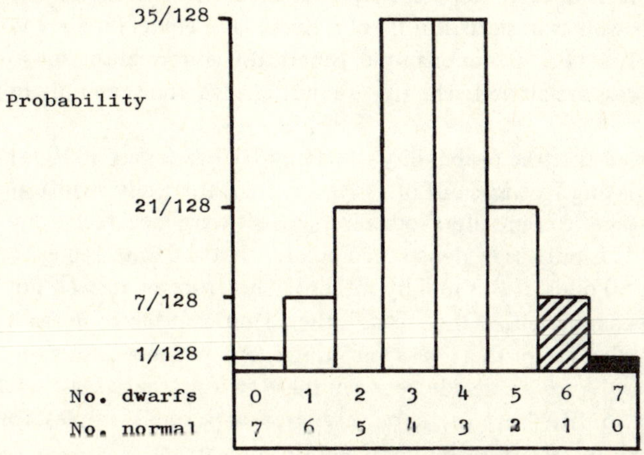

Fig. 14 The probability of 0 - 7 dwarfs with 7 children if the odds for each dwarf are 50 : 50.

The total shaded area, for example, represents the value, 'p' of having a result as extreme in the one direction as 6 dwarfs out of 7. Remember 'p' includes not only a result being as extreme as the one observed but also includes the probability of a more extreme result. Hence 'p', for at least 6 out of 7 dwarfs, assuming the null hypothesis is true, $\frac{7}{128} + \frac{1}{128} = \frac{8}{128} = \frac{1}{16} =$ (0,0625) which is not statistically significant even at the 0,05 level. The shaded area in the diagram (Figure 14) does not consider the probability of the equally extreme outcome at the other end of the scale - the probability of one or no dwarfs. Figure 14 shows that the probability of the bishop and the actress having no dwarfs out of 7 children is the same mathematically as that of having all 7 dwarfs. Is this outcome to be included in the estimate 'p' in significance tests? Both extremes are considered in what is called two tailed tests but not in one tailed tests.

Examples where one tailed tests (you sometimes see comments to this effect in the journals) may be used in medical practice are
1. if previous work suggests an outcome, e.g. do children with bilharzia score *lower* on I.Q. tests - we know they do not score higher.
2. if satisfied with an older and *cheaper* drug you may only be interested in whether a new one is better.

The use of a one tailed test has the effect of lowering the value of 'p' without altering the size of the sample (Figure 14) because in a two tailed test the 'p' value is twice what it is in a one tailed test.

Of course, as an aside, it must be stated that whether or not previous children are dwarfs does not alter the risks for subsequent children. This is so in genetic as well as in statistical theory. Some lay people, (and medical) think that if a first child is, for example, genetically abnormal the subsequent chances of success are altered. The risks do not change - one can only hope that luck will.

Table 8 showed that the probability of having 10 dwarfs out of 10 is more extreme than having 7 dwarfs out of 7; 10 is more statistically significant. Of course the genetic counsellors' odds if incorrect were incorrect from the beginning. It is only as evidence accumulates that the time comes to reject the 50 : 50 odds of this null hypothesis. Therefore an answer 'not significant' means that either there is no other significant factor in reality or if there is such a factor there is as yet insufficient evidence for us to accept it. The only way to decide between these two alternatives is to take a larger sample. A difference has to be very large, with small samples, for us to conclude it is a statistically significant difference.

The second last category of mistakes mentioned in Table 1 was 'negative conclusions being incorrectly stated'. It is wrong with negative results to state categorically that a nonsignificant difference means that there is definitely no difference at all. 'Dogmatism is puppyism come to its full growth' and it never pays to be too dogmatic that a difference does not exist. When a person concludes wrongly but justifiably on the evidence of the 'p' value that a difference does not exist, statisticians call this a Type II error.

Nor can we ever prove a difference does exist. Statistically a Type I error is where we reject the null hypothesis on the mathematical evidence and accept that some real factor is causing an effect when in fact the observed difference is only due to chance. The genetic counsellors may have given correct odds all the time. Even after 15 consecutive dwarfs when 'p'$\lll$0,001 and the probability of such a result occuring by chance is markedly less than 1 in 30 000, even then these results *could* still be just due to chance.

Another common category of mistakes was 'positive conclusions being incorrectly stated'. For example we read that 'without doubt' a difference existed - a positive finding incorrectly stated. Others calculated that 'p' was say 0,05 and then said they were 95 per cent convinced that a real difference existed - in fact they were 5 per cent unconvinced.

William Murray said, 'Give your decisions but never your reasons. Your decisions may be right but your reasons are sure to be wrong'. If we could be wrong all the time you may be wondering about the purpose of significance tests. The Type I and Type II errors are important and it is wise to know they exist, but we should not let them rule the roost. The significance levels let us off the hook. Even if really we are only becoming more and more doubtful of the Null Hypothesis as 'p' diminishes, by measuring this doubt against yardsticks in significance tests, we are able to distinguish between 'I am prepared to believe' and 'I am *not* prepared to believe'. Unless we can make such a decision we are not likely to be able to decide about a course of action and a significant result requires action and 'more persons on the whole are humbugged by believing nothing than by believing too much'.

To summarise, then, a signicicance test is like a trial in law. The victim is the Null Hypothesis who always pleads not guilty. We give him a fair trial, I hope, with random samples and meaningful control groups. The strength of his defence is measured by 'p' and we listen, withdraw, and weigh up the evidence using statistical tables before reaching a verdict.

If you like, if 'p'$<$0,05 we can give a fine as a sentence. If 'p'$<$0,01 we can put the Null Hypothesis in jail. We can even metaphorically hang the Null Hypothesis if 'p'$<$0,001. What we can never do is prove him guilty.

There are five side issues in making any trial fair. Firstly, if one intends to act on the result it is probably better to select one significance level in particular before one starts. Secondly, beware of the author who uses lots of tests on the same results! This was the least common category of mistakes in the journal evaluation (Table 1). Remember that, using the 0,05 significance level, one would expect a statistically significant difference with no real effect, in one out of every twenty tests. It is possible, but not usually desirable, to carry out many tests, but allowance has to be made for this in assessing 'p'. Thirdly, remember that the sample size has been taken into account in calculating 'p'. It is therefore wrong to say that 'the difference is statistically significant and moreover a very big sample was taken' as though this adds more weight to the argument. If anything, it detracts, because the smaller the sample the larger the difference has to be to attain statistical significance.

Fourthly, the results may be very highly significant statistically but one must ask oneself whether the comparisons are meaningful from other points of view. Is the control group correct? Are we comparing people of different genetic backgrounds and attributing their differences to diet? Fifthly, do not confuse statistical significance with practical importance - an importand distinction both in designing your own research and in interpreting the answers of others.

10. So what?

Have you had the measles?
If so how many?
Armstrong Ward

This last point in the previous chapter is one for which statistics and statisticians cannot be blamed. It seems to me that there is a tendency among editors of medical journals to confuse 'statistical significance' with 'practical importance'. At the end of an analysis one is often tempted to say, 'So what?' If information is not important, no matter how significant the difference, I would join in the chorus with other practising doctors by saying 'So what?'

This is the age of technology and numbers. The least we can do in medical research is to assign a meaningful figure to the results - to the meaningful results of practical importance, I hope.

If the findings are of medical importance they ought to be brought to the attention of other jockeys in the same race:

It takes two to speak the truth -
One to speak and another to hear.
H.D. Thoreau.

The grammatical part of an article does not usually concern me because my own English is not very good. But as Winston Churchill said, 'This is the sort of English up with which I will not put' , and words like 'probable', 'significant'. 'random' and 'unbiased' are words which have special statistical implications and in a scientific project they should not, I feel, be used unscientifically.

My overall four conclusions for the medical research worker are these.

Firstly, make sure there is a practical implication in the work you intend to undertake. Secondly, plan before you start. Spell out the question, decide on what measurements are needed, who will measure and whom they will measure, how the results will be presented, how they will be analysed and interpreted and only then start the actual research. My third piece of advice is to stick to the simple things of life and above all be honest. In this numbers game we want the truth, the whole truth and nothing but the truth.

In this book I have taken the liberty of criticising the editors of medical journals for publishing articles which contained too many errors. Many of these errors were caused by a lack of knowledge of statistics, how statistics can be put into operation, its limitations and many pitfalls.

To be completely honest I think the worst article ever published was written by myself and my late colleague, Dr D.A.W. Rittey (he was not the ghost writer!). The editor of the Central African Journal, Professor Michael Gelfand, has given me permission to reproduce this article here.

The reference numbers indicate phrases or expression which we, the authors, contrived to introduce as being representative of the very errors which I have suggested in this book, should be avoided. As an exercise the reader may wish to 'spot the errors'. A key is provided in the list of references describing the errors as we saw them but I'm sure there are other errors undetected by the authors.

William Shakespeare said that 'some people would lie with such volubility that you would think truth were the fool'. Dr Rittey, who not only was learned but looked learned presented this paper once with a poker face at a local clinical meeting at which distinguished overseas medical academics were present. The paper provoked interesting discussion - about medical problems associated with African westernisation - not about the misuse of statistics in operation.

Revision exercise: An association between carbohydrate intake and the incidence of ulcerative colitis

Introduction

A recent survey from America (Snoopy, Module *et al*)[1] suggests that patients with ulcerative colitis are thinner than others.[2] In an attempt to follow up this finding[3] the authors carried out an experiment locally to confirm[4] that the disease was caused[5] by a low carbohydrate intake.

Method

A large team[6] of highly trained dieticians closely questioned[7] 1 000[8] hospital admissions,[9] 500 Europeans and 500 Africans. This was to determine the average difference between the carbohydrate intake of the two racial groups.[10] The questioners were particularly interested in the findings that with the Africans as the percentage of carbohydrate intake[11] increased so the percentage of protein intake decreased.[12] (See Figure 1.)[13]

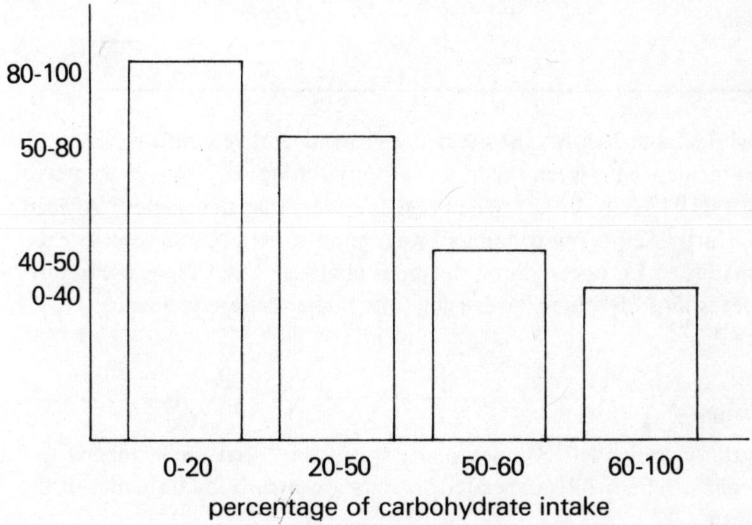

Fig. 1 The relationship between carbohydrate and protein uptake in the 500 Africans. The fat and alcohol intake are excluded

They report that this may indicate a need for health education.[14]

Results

Table 1 The carbohydrate intake in the two groups

	More than 50%	Less than 50%	
African	409	91	498
Europeans	263	234	497
	670	325	995

180 per cent more Europeans than Africans appreciate the value of a low carbohydrate diet!

Table 1[15] above shows the 995[16] patients grouped by race and whether they consumed more-or-less than 50 per cent carbohydrate in their diet.[17] These results proved without doubt[18] that Europeans eat less carbohydrate[19] than the Africans ('p'>001).[20]

Table 2 Cases of ulcerative colitis in the two groups

	Ulcerative Colitis	Other Diagnoses	
African	1	469	470
European	27	455	482
	28	924	952

Meanwhile Table 2 shows the incidence[21] of ulcerative colitis.[22] The difference in incidence between the hypo-carbohydrating Africans is very nearly significant. 057 (c.f. .05).[24] When one considers that the single[25] African case on further close questioning[26] was found to be a school teacher eating a mainly[27] European diet it becomes obvious[28] that the low carbohydrate diet is most definitely[18] causing[5] the higher disease incidence[21] (Figure 2.)[29]

Discussion

This strictly controlled[10] experiment[30] confirms[4] that the incidence[21] difference can be firmly associated[5] with a lower carbohydrate diet of the European.

It is true that for the purpose of weight accretion[23] there might be variations in daily carbohydration[23] by the Europeans but these fall well within recognised parameters.[23] It is very significant[28] that the only African case was a school teacher on a hyperproteinised diet.[31] This confirms the view of Soap, J.[1] (1968) who, in a controlled study of ulcerative colitis in urbanised Eskimos and rural aborigines[10] concluded that a hypercarbohydration programme is valueless without a concomitant hyper-proteinisation diet with penicillinisation[23] of the intestinal flora affecting endoabsorption.[23]

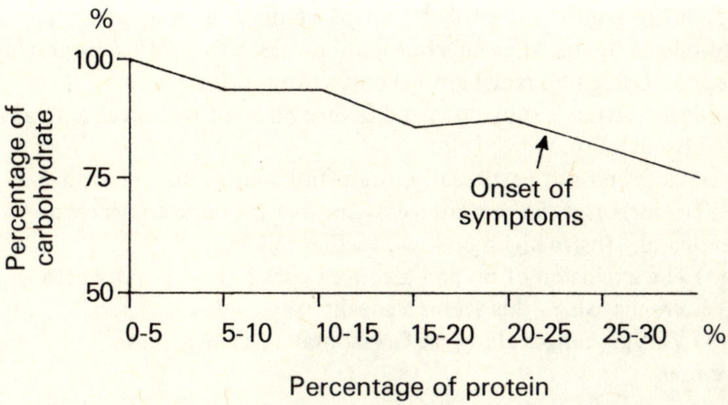

Fig. 2 Assessment of percentage carbohydrate

The authors report that they themselves intend to carry out further experiments[30] to determine whether a high carbohydrate diet protects the African or the low carbohydrate diet causes the disease in the Europeans.[32]

Conclusion

Good medical punters would agree with the majority of these references and could, no doubt, add more.

References

1. An international reputation does not guarantee the worthiness of the comment.
2. 'Others' ought to be defined.
3. In fact it is a suggestion and unless it is more clearly defined it is impossible to 'follow up'.
4. 'Confirm' suggests that the local authors have already decided what the answer is. Suspect them of bias.
5. The authors are probably mistakenly thinking that association and causation are synonymous; statistics help us to test association but not causation Remember lung cancer is *associated* with smoking; it does not *cause* people to smoke!

6. The larger the team the greater the variation in interpretation of results. It is generally better to limit the number of observers.
7. The answers to questions are subjective and very liable to bias.
8. A large sample cannot correct badly designed research.
9. Hospital admission should be more closely defined. Are maternity cases and paediatric cases included, for example? Moreover, hospital admissions are notoriously unreliable.
10. Wrong control group - the correct control would be a group as similar as possible to one of the racial groups but without ulcerative colitis, preferably not in hospital. Using two racial groups only confuses the issue.
11. Dietary information is subjective and is very difficult to collect with any semblance of reliability.
12. It is inevitable and not particularly interesting that as the precentage of one ingredient increases the percentage of another is bound to decrease.
13. This misleading figure highlights two further points:

(a) The exclusion of fat and alcohol seems to be a point worth emphasising - this seems a sneaky way of doing this.

(b) Varying ranges along the horizontal axis can mislead.

Locum wanted!!

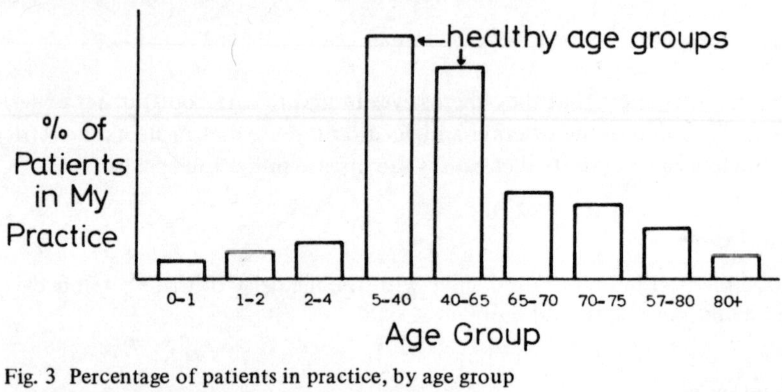

Fig. 3 Percentage of patients in practice, by age group

Minimal paediatrics and geriatrics with consequently very few night calls.
14. Journalistic asides are unwarranted in a scientific description of a method.
15. Besides the arithmetical errors in this table the conclusion is stated in an unnecessary 'loaded' fashion. Also
16. There are 'missing results' not accounted for. Are they perhaps ulcerative colitis patients on a high carbohydrate diet? We need to know whether their absence is related to the topic under discussion.
17. See 11. The original (quantitative) measurement is more valuable than this (qualitative) dichotomy.
18. Statistics never 'prove without doubt' but measure doubt.

19.We have no information yet about the *actual amount* of carbohydrate.
20.Presumably p .001 is the conclusion. As it stands p could be any value, e.g. 0,99.
21.Incidence is the term answering the question 'how often?' The term prevalence required here answers the question 'how common?'.
22.The disease has not been defined fully. The criteria of diagnosis must be mentioned.
23.There is no need for 'hyper-intellectual' words.
24.The purpose of the significance level 0,05 is to enable us to decide whether we conclude that results are either significant or not significant. There is no such conclusion as 'nearly significant' particularly when it is 'very nearly significant'.
25.Signle is an ambiguous word. Is he unmarried or is he 'the one'?
26.See 7. It is inconceivable that 'further close questioning' is needed to reveal the type of diet when the patient has already been 'closely questioned'. This suggests that all the original replies are unreliable.
27.Words like 'mainly' are very subjective. I think one deserves to be told exactly what this patient eats especially as
28.His presence is so important to the author's case. He has already been included once in the analysis, and to mention him again 50 times does not cause the results to 'become obvious'. Remember, one is not yet aware whether he eats more-or-less than 50 per cent carbohydrate - perhaps his mainly European diet is sandwiches for lunch and cakes for tea!
29.A graph from one person! It is rather sneaky not to show the zero. Both axes are related (13a).
30.This 'experiment' is a 'survey'. This means that a significant result could be due to chance, the factor under review or some associated factor - such as race!
31.This is not true. See Figure 2. In fact he seems to eat about 25 per cent protein and 75 per cent carbohydrate.
32.Well, well, well!

Glossary

Age Specific Mortality Rate	See Table 5 (page 64)
Cause Specific Mortality Rate	See Table 5 (page 64)
Correlation Coefficient	a measure of how closely more than one variable are associated
Crude Death Rate	See Table 5 (page 64)
Directly Standardised Rate	A standardised rate which different known age specific mortality rates are applied to a standard population
Incidence Rate	$\frac{\text{The number of cases of disease Y beginning in specified period x 1 000}}{\text{Average number of persons in that population in that period}}$
Indirectly Standardised Rate	A standardised rate in which standard age specific mortality rates are applied to different known populations.
Infant Mortality Rate	See Table 5 (page 65)
Life Expectancy ($^{o}e_{x}$)	The average length of subsequent life lived by those attaining their xth birthday
Maternal Mortality Rate	See Table 5 (page 64)
Mean	The arithmetical average of the results
Median	Middle results when the results are ranked = 50th percentile
Mode	Most frequent result
Neonatal Mortality Rate	See Table 5 (page 65)
Percentage	The proportion multiplied by 100
Percentile	The percentage of results lying below a particular result
Perinatal Mortality Rate	See Table 5 (page 65)
Period Prevalence	$\frac{\text{The number of cases of disease Y existing in specified period x 1 000}}{\text{Average number of persons in that population in that period}}$

Point Prevalence	$\frac{\text{The number of cases of disease Y existing at specified time x 1 000}}{\text{Number of persons in that population at that time}}$
Proportion	The number observed with a characteristic divided by the total
Range	The difference between the largest and the smallest result
Ratio	The number observed with a characteristic divided by the number without that characteristic
*Regression Coefficient (*linear*)*	The average rate at which one variable increases in association with another
Standard Deviation	The square root of the variance
*Standard Error (*of mean*)*	The standard deviation of means of random samples of a given size (N) from a given population which equals the standard deviation of the primary data divided by the square root of the number in the sample
Standardised Mortality Rate	The ratio of actual deaths observed to those which would be expected from applying age specific death rates from a standard population
Post Neonatal Mortality Rate	See Table 5 (page 65)
Standard Rate	A rate adjusted to refer to a standard or typical population
Stillbirth Rate	See Table 5 (page 64)
Variance	The sum of the squares of the deviations from the mean divided by 1 less than the number of observations.

Further Reading

Armitage, P.	(1973)	*Statistical Methods in Medical Research,* 2nd edn., Blackwell, Oxford.
Bailey, N.T.J.	(1959)	*Statistical Methods in Biology,* English Universities Press.
Benjamin, B.	(1968)	*Health and Vital Statistics,* George Allen and Unwin, London.
Bourke, G.J. & McGilvry, J.	(1975)	*Interpretation and Uses of Medical Statistics,* 2nd edn., Blackwell, Oxford.
Castle, W.M.	(1977)	*Statistics in Small Doses,* 2nd edn., Churchill Livingstone, Edinburgh.
Cox, D.R.	(1958)	*Planning of Experiments,* Wiley, London.
England, J.M.	(1975)	*Medical Research, a Statistical and Epidemiological Approach,* Churchill Livingstone, Edinburgh.
Hill, A. Bradford	(1971)	*Principles of Medical Statistics,* 9th edn., The Lancet, London.
Hills, M.	(1974)	*Statistics for Comparative Studies,* Chapman & Hall.
Maxwell, A.E.	(1961)	*Analysing Qualitative Data,* Methuen & Co. Ltd., London.
Maxwell, C.	(1973)	*Clinical Research for All,* Cambridge Medical Publications.

Index